Theraplay®
Theory, Applications and Implementation

Theraplay®

Theory, Applications and Implementation

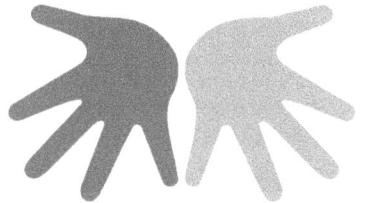

Edited by
Sandra Lindaman and **Rana Hong**

Foreword by **Phyllis Booth**

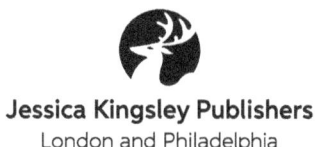

Jessica Kingsley Publishers
London and Philadelphia

First published in Great Britain in 2021 by Jessica Kingsley Publishers
An Hachette Company

1

Copyright © Jessica Kingsley Publishers 2021
Foreword copyright © Phyllis Booth 2021

A CIP catalogue record for this title is available from the
British Library and the Library of Congress

ISBN 978 1 78775 070 8
eISBN 978 1 78775 071 5

Printed and bound in the United States by Integrated Books International

Jessica Kingsley Publishers' policy is to use papers that are natural,
renewable and recyclable products and made from wood grown in
sustainable forests. The logging and manufacturing processes are expected
to conform to the environmental regulations of the country of origin.

Jessica Kingsley Publishers
73 Collier Street
London N1 9BE, UK

www.jkp.com

Contents

Foreword

Theraplay began in the late 1960s as a creative response to a challenging situation. The approach was timely in meeting the needs of preschoolers in the citywide Chicago Head Start program. In many ways, it was ahead of its time in applying new ideas about attachment to child treatment. Because Theraplay is modeled on basic parent-child relationships, it is also timeless. To understand where Theraplay is today, we should remind ourselves of where it came from and how it has developed over the years.

In 1967, Ann Jernberg was given the assignment to provide psychological services for all the Head Start programs in Chicago. She recruited a group of people who had experience working with children. Since Ann and I had been nursery school teachers together some years before, she asked me to join her team. Our mandate was to identify children in need of psychological services and then refer them to existing child treatment centers. In order to do this, we consulted with the teachers and observed the children in their classrooms. The children we identified fell roughly into two groups: those who were angry, acting out and difficult to manage, and those who were fearful, withdrawn or frozen and unable to participate in the program. We had expected the teachers to identify the acting-out children more than the withdrawn ones because they present a bigger problem in managing the classroom. But we found that the teachers were equally likely to identify quiet, withdrawn children as needing help. As we understand it now, the common thread between the two groups was that they did not feel safe enough to relax and enjoy the classroom experience. By the end of the first summer, we had identified more than 200 children who needed help. However, in Chicago, there were no treatment centers that were prepared to treat that many preschool children.

Faced with the challenge of finding no treatment available, Ann came up with her creative and audacious plan. We would recruit and train lively, engaging young people to go into the schools and work one on one with each child who needed help. In order to identify the applicants who were most likely to be successful with the children, we held group recruiting days at the Theraplay office. We asked the applicants to role-play with a partner how they might interact with a four-year-old child in a session. From each group of applicants, we chose those who were the most engaging, lively and responsive with their "child" partner. If Stephen Porges, creator of polyvagal theory (2011), had been there to give us the language, we would have said that we chose those who were most able to use their social engagement system to create a sense of safety, acceptance and shared fun.

We instructed our new recruits to engage each child assigned to them in the way that good enough parents interact with their young children: sensitively, spontaneously, face to face, with no need for toys, simply inviting the child to join them in joyful, interactive play. Our goal was to create a relationship of trust and safety between child and practitioner. In weekly supervisory sessions, we helped our practitioners reflect on their own and the child's experience in order to be more attuned to each child's needs. Together we came up with new activities that we could use to engage and delight the children as well as to calm and comfort them. We saw each child two or three times a week and averaged about 15 sessions per child. We were soon delighted with our results: angry, aggressive, acting-out children calmed down and were able to engage with others in a friendly, cooperative way; sad, withdrawn children became livelier and more outgoing.

Our playful, interactive approach ran counter to the then typical patterns of child therapy and we faced considerable opposition from traditionally trained social workers and therapists. To meet their opposition Ann made two films, *Here I Am* (1969) and *There He Goes* (1975), as examples of successful Theraplay treatment. In the first film, a withdrawn, mute and immobile girl is helped by the challenge of age-appropriate expectations and direct engagement. In the second film, an extremely active, aggressive and rejecting boy, a "tough guy…with a hungry baby inside" (as described in the film), is helped by additional structure and nurture.

How could we understand and explain to ourselves and others what made our approach so effective? The first step in my personal understanding came out of my experience in 1969–70 at the Tavistock Centre in London studying with John Bowlby and Donald Winnicott. Bowlby's first book about attachment was published at that time (Bowlby, 1969).

When I returned to Chicago in the fall of 1970, Ann showed me her first film, along with the newly constructed Theraplay room. It was a large, uncluttered room with mats on the floor and a lot of wonderful big pillows—a room that invited the face-to-face, interactive play that was proving so helpful to the Head Start children. There were two observation rooms with one-way mirrors and equipment for filming the sessions that took place there.

I was immediately on board with the exciting new project of working with the Head Start children. I found myself making use of what I had learned in London to help me understand why using the model of healthy parenting was making a difference. I remember saying to Ann, "We are creating Winnicott's 'Holding environment.'" I was referring to his belief that devoted mothers create a sense of safety and acceptance—a nurturing world where the child can thrive. From Winnicott, I also learned the importance of "being present" as we interacted with the children. I attended a lecture he gave to young psychoanalysts in training in which he advised them to not try to come up with clever interpretations, but rather to just *be there* with their patients (Personal communication, 1970).

From Bowlby, I understood the importance of the parent-child model that we were using. In 1953, he had written, "The quality of the parental care which a child receives in his earliest years is of vital importance for his future mental health" (Bowlby, 1953, p.11). In writing about Theraplay in 1979, Ann reaffirmed her original focus: "The best way to understand the principles underlying the Theraplay method is to rediscover the basics of the mother-infant relationship" (Jernberg, 1979, p.4). She traced "Theraplay principles to the mother-infant nursery day—particularly those intimate, empathic, playful parts of the day that evoke competence, trust and joy" (p.xii). She believed that "'understood infants', in contrast to those who missed out on early empathic understanding, should be less likely to manifest profound psychological damage later" (p.16). In his 1988 book, Bowlby said much the same thing: "The pattern of interaction adopted by the mother of a secure infant provides an excellent model for the pattern of therapeutic intervention" (Bowlby, 1988, p.126).

Another step in our understanding of what made our work successful came from Bowlby's idea that the patterns of interaction between a child and a caregiver create internal working models for the child. We felt that the dyadic experience of feeling safe and being sensitively responded to, validated and enjoyed had created a new and more positive internal working model for each child. In the first Theraplay book, Ann quotes me as saying, "The child must come to see, reflected in the therapist's eyes, the image of himself both as lovable and as fun to be with" (Jernberg, 1979, p.3). And of course our ultimate goal is that the parents become this important presence, defining and reflecting the child's positive sense of self.

As I look back on this history, I realize that in many ways we were ahead of our time in exploring ways to incorporate attachment theory into our model. During the past 50 years, attachment theory has spawned a great deal of research into the nature of the caregiver-infant relationship and its effect on the child's mind; many therapeutic approaches now incorporate these concepts in their work. This research has enabled us to understand more about what is actually happening in the healthy caregiver-child relationship and thus helped us fine-tune our work. I am confident that more insights will follow as people continue to study aspects of what goes on in the early caregiver-child relationship.

While our initial understanding of what made our work effective came from Bowlby and Winnicott's ideas about the importance of the mother-child relationship, Theraplay also integrated ideas from a variety of other sources. Ann describes the roots of Theraplay as found "in psychoanalysis, developmental psychology, and nursery school practice, it is not so much a break with tradition as it is a gleaning from a number of fields" (1979, p.xi).

Currently, the contribution of the therapist and therapeutic presence is considered a critical factor in the therapy process leading to change. Theraplay has always valued the therapist's presence, describing the therapist as the most important "object" in the playroom. Being able to reflect on our own and others' emotional experience is now seen as an important capacity, making it possible for parents and therapist to respond in the sensitive, attuned manner that leads to secure attachment. Reflective supervision is now considered best practice as well. From the very beginning, it has been essential to our work that we reflect on our own experience and that of the child. We provided reflective supervision to our Head Start mental health workers, helping them understand the child's experience as well as their own emotional responses. Filming sessions in our private clinic made it possible for us to review our work and learn more about the child's reactions as well as our own responses. Reviewing films of the Marschak Interaction Method for parents and children helped us fine-tune our understanding of the relationship between parent and child, and identify areas of strengths to build on and areas in which they needed help. We were able to use the film during feedback sessions with parents to help them reflect on their own and their child's feelings and responses.

We have also been very aware of the need to understand our own countertransference issues. In the final chapter of the first Theraplay book, Ann discusses the hazards of acting out in the countertransference and suggests ways to monitor and control such actions (1979, pp.431–436). The therapist's use of self as a critical part of the Theraplay model will be discussed in Chapter 1 and throughout this book.

Over the 50 years since Theraplay began, it has reflected and responded to the special needs and issues of the time. The first need, of course, was to help the Head Start children. When we began seeing families in The Theraplay Institute playroom, Ann noted that a popular style of extremely democratic parenting created burdens for children. The preface to her 1979 book begins with the scene of a three-year-old child asking and then pleading with her parents to tell her whether it might rain and whether she should put her boots on. Because they want to foster her independence and autonomy, the parents refuse to answer. Recognizing the child's pain, Ann intervenes: "It's going to rain, Clarissa. Put your boots on." The child is calmed and happily puts her boots on for the walk.

Ann believed that this "democratic" approach left children feeling unsafe and anxious. Because no one else was willing to take a guiding role, the children became what she called "Little Tyrants," taking charge and "calling all the shots." The goal of Theraplay for such families was to help parents provide clear guidance and structure that would create a sense of safety for the child. In the 1980s, Jernberg was featured in *Newsweek* magazine speaking against a new parenting trend that created "super babies." She advised play as an antidote to the pressure to perform that parents and children were feeling. Beginning in the 1990s, Theraplay helped parents of internationally adopted children to understand the effects of loss, institutional care and trauma on the development of a new parent-child attachment. Now a greater understanding of the impact of childhood adversity lights the way for the use of Theraplay as a trauma-informed model of care for prevention and amelioration of the effects of adverse childhood events. Chapters in this book will address this issue. Additionally, Theraplay is well prepared to respond to the developmental threats posed by the current electronic and social media age with its lack of face-to-face interaction and physical, active play.

In addition to being both ahead of its time and timely, Theraplay principles are timeless in that they are based on the universal experience of parent-child care and interaction which, when it goes well, supports the development of the capacity to relate, to regulate, to learn acceptable ways of interacting and to become a successfully functioning adult. Since these patterns vary from culture to culture, it is essential that we, as practitioners, be open to understanding the parenting patterns and acceptable behavior within the culture of the families with whom we work.

As I have said, Theraplay began as a response to a challenge 50 years ago. During that time, Theraplay practitioners have faced new challenges and come up with innovative responses. Each chapter in this book describes an adaptation of Theraplay to a specific need. The chapters include detailed suggestions for readers about how to apply the insights and experience of the writers, along with treatment vignettes illustrating the process.

Chapter 1 provides an overview of the protocol, dimensions and goals of Theraplay. Four critical Theraplay processes are discussed and illustrated with case examples: establishing safety and arousal regulation, enhancing caregiver-child attachment, working with parents in and out of session, and the Theraplay practitioner's use of self.

Chapter 2 explores the question of why some parents, while clearly invested in helping their child, seem unable to shift the behaviors that are contributing to the family cycle. Before we can achieve the goal of healing the relationship with their child, we must fully understand the parent's experience and help them to feel heard and understood. The author tells us how to use the information from the Adult Attachment Interview questions in order to understand—and help parents understand—how their experiences affect their relationship with their child.

Chapter 3 describes the use of Theraplay prenatally and with infants and toddlers. Since Theraplay is modeled on the healthy parent-child interaction, it is an obvious choice to be used in this way to strengthen the emotional bond between parent and child. This chapter presents a structured program designed to enhance early emotional attachment, beginning during pregnancy and extending into the early months of the baby's life. The authors report on their research confirming the beneficial effects of the program with a group of depressed and troubled mothers.

Chapter 4 addresses the question of why we would use a treatment based on the model of parents and young children when working with an adolescent. It presents a convincing argument for adapting Theraplay to help adolescents successfully navigate this confusing time of their life. The lively examples of Theraplay interaction with families and groups paint a clear and compelling picture of how the work can be done.

Chapter 5 describes how Theraplay-based Sunshine Circles are used in classrooms to support the social-emotional development of young children. Sunshine Circles create a sense of safety and connection within the classroom as well as helping children regulate, relax and learn. The case illustration provides a lively view of a successful course of Sunshine Circles in a Head Start program.

Chapter 6 outlines the values and challenges of doing Theraplay in the family home. Home-based Theraplay makes it possible to bring Theraplay to families who are not able to come to a conventional therapy office setting. It also makes it easier to support the ongoing use of Theraplay ideas and philosophy within the home setting. The author describes the important considerations and adaptations required to make home-based Theraplay successful.

Chapter 7 describes Theraplay as an ideal intervention for anxiety because it establishes a more secure, authoritative caregiver-child relationship. Additionally, Theraplay attends to the needs of both caregiver and child, which is helpful because anxiety is often intergenerational. The chapter gives specific dimension- and treatment-phase-related examples of increasing predictability and role definition.

Chapter 8 describes how Theraplay contributes to the treatment and healing of children who have suffered sexual abuse: by developing emotional and behavioral co-regulation; establishing or re-establishing a more secure attachment; creating relational boundaries, including the safe and healthy use of touch; prioritizing the child's developmental needs; and empowering and improving self-esteem.

Chapter 9 describes the "By Your Side Model," which uses Theraplay to support a successful transition from foster care to adoption. The child's current foster parents are included in Theraplay sessions along with the new adoptive caregivers. This makes it possible for the foster parents to share their views of the child with the new family as well as to provide a bridge of safety and care as the child makes this difficult transition.

Chapter 10 describes how Theraplay can be used to help families affected by domestic violence. The chapter gives the reader essential information about domestic violence and its impact on the caregiver and child. The first phase of treatment is working with the non-offending caregiver to establish that caregiver's sense of safety, regulation and empowerment. The chapter gives clear and lively explanations for how to use the dimensions of Theraplay during the dyadic work to give specific, helpful messages to the caregiver and child to counteract the trauma of domestic violence.

Chapter 11 describes how to adapt Theraplay for affirmative intervention with lesbian, gay, bisexual, transgender and queer (LGBTQ) families. The author helps Theraplay practitioners understand the impact of LGBTQ-related stigma on attachment bonds, how LGBTQ affirmative language is critical to promote feelings of safety and worth, and how the Theraplay dimensions of nurture and engagement communicate unconditional love to the LGBTQ child/youth.

Chapter 12 introduces us to Theraplay with children who are deaf or hard of hearing. The chapter includes suggestions for how to make use of the non-verbal aspects of Theraplay to create a relationship, a sense of safety, and to convey to the child that the practitioner and the caregiver understand and can connect with them. The chapter explains the importance of knowing how those with hearing loss and their family members identify themselves, possible caregiver grief and loss reactions that can interfere with attachment, and how Theraplay is an ideal intervention when there are differences in the language systems of caregiver and child.

I want to express my admiration for the authors and my deep gratitude for the contribution that they have made to Theraplay by sharing their expertise with us. These authors clearly are dedicated to their clients and to finding solutions for difficult problems. I also want to thank readers for your interest in Theraplay, whether you are new to Theraplay or have taken a Theraplay training or are in our supervision process. It makes me very happy and hopeful that the Theraplay I have loved and nurtured for 50 years is also treasured by younger practitioners in many countries. Your interest makes me confident that Theraplay will continue to help families for many more years.

Phyllis Booth

References

Bowlby, J. (1953). *Child Care and the Growth of Love*. London, UK: Penguin Books.

Bowlby, J. (1969). *Attachment. Attachment and Loss (vol 1)* (first edition). London, UK: The Hogarth Press.

Bowlby, J. (1988). *A Secure Base: Parent-Child Attachment and Healthy Human Development*. New York, NY: Basic Books.

Jernberg, A.M. (1979). *Theraplay*. San Francisco, CA: Jossey-Bass Publishers.

Porges, S.W. (2011). *The Polyvagal Theory: Neurophysiological Foundations of Emotions, Attachment, Communication, and Self-Regulation*. New York, NY: W.W. Norton & Company.

Acknowledgments

Thanks to my husband Ken for his support and nurture.

Thanks to Phyllis Booth for her wisdom and friendship.

Thanks to the authors of this book for their passion for Theraplay and their compassion for families.

Thanks to my colleagues around the world for their embrace of Theraplay.

Sandra Lindaman

I thank my family for their loving support and care. I feel blessed to have my son, Daniel, for his expressed sensitivity by bringing me cups of coffee on many late nights. I thank my best friend, Seyoung Kim, for her constant encouragement and friendship. Most importantly, a special appreciation goes to the authors of this book for sharing their invaluable experience to advance Theraplay.

Rana Hong

Preface

The goal of Theraplay has always been to establish a healthy emotional connection between child and caregiver. Now, in the current times, in the face of coronavirus and the COVID-19 pandemic, children more than ever need to feel safe and connected to their primary caregivers. A positive child-caregiver relationship is the foundation of a moment to moment and lifelong sense of safety and emotional health. Theraplay achieves this by providing new experiences of positive social engagement, reciprocity, play, pleasure, joy and soothing care. Typically, the Theraplay practitioner takes an active role in initiating interactions with the child and caregiver, and gradually transitions to child-caregiver interaction. The chapters in this book were written before the pandemic and describe steps in the typical Theraplay model. As we write this preface, Theraplay practitioners are creating new ways to convey the positive experiences of Theraplay via telehealth parent-child interaction assessment, parent preparation and guidance of parent-child play sessions. Theraplay practitioners in some places in the world are even conducting Sunshine Circles with groups of children, each in their own home, via digital platforms! Our in-person way of delivering Theraplay may be altered for a short or long while, but the goals and basic tools remain the same as described in this book. Theraplay continues to be a way to come together in the face of gaps in human connection. What is essential is that we find our way to create connection because we know that relationships heal.

Sandra Lindaman and Rana Hong
May 30, 2020

The Authors

Editors

Sandra Lindaman, MA, MSW, LCSW, LISW-CP is a Certified Theraplay® Practitioner, Supervisor and Trainer, and the Senior Training Advisor for The Theraplay Institute in Evanston, Illinois, USA. Sandra has been with The Theraplay Institute since 1990 and was Executive Director from 1993 to 1999. She learned how to do Theraplay by serving as a co-therapist with Phyllis Booth while Ann Jernberg worked with the parents. She co-authored three chapters in the 2010 third edition of *Theraplay: Helping Parents and Children Build Better Relationships Through Attachment-Based Play*. Sandra has published other chapters and journal articles about attachment, adoption, reunification, selective mutism, autism, play therapy and the neuroscience foundation of the Theraplay model. Sandra has been very involved in Theraplay training curriculum development and the training and supervision of professionals in the Theraplay model throughout the United States, Canada, UK, Denmark, Finland, Sweden, Japan, South Korea and Hong Kong. In 2004, she received the Ann M. Jernberg award for outstanding contribution to Theraplay.

Rana Hong, PhD, MSW, LCSW, RPT-S is a Certified Theraplay® Practitioner, Supervisor and Trainer and President of the Board of Directors for The Theraplay Institute in Evanston, Illinois, USA. Rana is a Research Assistant Professor at Loyola University Chicago School of Social Work and a therapist in private practice in Des Plaines, Illinois. She has incorporated Theraplay as one of her core treatment models since 2001. With her clinical expertise in attachment and trauma-based models, Rana is committed to enhancing the psychological self-sufficiency of clients. Exemplars of Rana's recent publications are "Neurobiological core content in the research supported Transforming Impossible into

Possible program model" (2019), "Utilizing clinical theory to understand psychological self-sufficiency" (2019) and "Becoming a neurobiologically informed play therapist" (2016).

Contributing authors

Karen Doyle Buckwalter, MSW, LCSW, RPT-S is a Certified Theraplay® Practitioner, Supervisor and Trainer, and the Director of Program Strategy, Chaddock in Quincy, Illinois, USA. Karen has a research and clinical interest in the intergenerational transmission of attachment as assessed by the Adult Attachment Interview (AAI); she completed the intensive AAI training at the Attachment and Human Development Center in Washington, DC, in 2008. She has since reviewed over 150 coded AAI interviews with Dr. Miriam Steele, focused on the clinical application of AAI data when working with highly distressed adoption dyads. Karen is trained in other dyadic models of therapy including child-parent psychotherapy with Alicia Lieberman and Patricia Van Horn. Karen co-edited *Attachment Theory in Action* (2018) and co-authored *Raising the Challenging Child* (2020).

Donna M. Gates, MA, LCPC is a Certified Theraplay® Practitioner, Supervisor and Trainer. She is a Senior Supervisor at The Theraplay Institute, supervising students in the Practitioner Practicum and candidates in the Supervisor Practicum. Donna has more than 25 years of clinical experience in family therapy, both in private practice and in a community youth and family agency. She has specialty training and experience in domestic violence (DV), having worked both with families who experience DV and with DV treatment groups for offenders. She has authored two articles on the use of Theraplay in DV treatment.

Eliana Gil, PhD, LMFT, RPT-S, ATR is the Senior Clinical Consultant at the Gil Institute for Trauma Recovery and Education, Fairfax, Virginia, USA. Eliana has more than 40 years' experience of working in the field of child abuse prevention and treatment. She has articulated an integrated clinical approach in order to help traumatized children and their families that includes expressive therapies with kinesthetic, sensory and brain-based approaches. Currently, Eliana teaches, consults and supervises. She is an Intermediate Level Theraplay practitioner and highly values

Theraplay, not only for its powerful dyadic approach but also because it provides dimensions of family interactions that help clinicians assess and target specific problem areas in the parent-child relationship.

Alexis Greeves, MA, LPCC, RPT-S is a Certified Theraplay® Practitioner and Trainer in private practice in the Twin Cities, Minneapolis, USA. Alexis teaches play therapy courses for graduate programs at Bethel University in St Paul, Minneapolis, and for Gallaudet University in Washington, DC, the only university for the Deaf in the world. While Alexis is herself a hearing person, she is proficient in American Sign Language and focuses her work on providing services to the Deaf community. She has found Theraplay to be an ideal intervention when the caregiver and child use different language systems.

Annie Kiermaier, LCSW, RN is a Certified Theraplay® Practitioner, Supervisor and Trainer. Annie has focused her professional work on strengthening attachments between children and their parents/caregivers, first as an obstetrical nurse and then as a clinical social worker specializing in home-based early intervention work in rural, coastal Maine. From 2013 to 2019, Annie spread many Theraplay "seeds" throughout the world as she led more than 150 training sessions. She hopes her chapter will inspire you to consider the benefits of home-based Theraplay, wherever you may be working with families.

Elizabeth Konrath, MA, LPC, RPT-S is a Certified Theraplay® Practitioner, Supervisor and Trainer. She is in private practice, seeing clients and supervising clinicians in Boulder, Colorado, USA. Before moving to Colorado, she had the privilege of working with Dr. Eliana Gil at the Gil Institute for Trauma Recovery and Education. Elizabeth spent five years in community mental health providing therapy for children in the foster care system in Washington, DC. She has extensive training in trauma, particularly working with children, adolescents and families whose lives are affected by physical abuse, sexual abuse, family violence, neglect, bullying and attachment issues related to adoption.

Hanna Lampi is an occupational therapist, a Certified Theraplay® Practitioner, Supervisor and Trainer and a family psychotherapist from Espoo, Finland. In her practice, she provides occupational therapy services for children and adolescents, Theraplay, family therapy and the Nurture and Play (NaP) intervention. She also teaches how to utilize the Theraplay and NaP frameworks in daycare, foster care and parenting programs. Hanna graduated from the Infant-Parent Mental Health Certificate program at the University of Massachusetts, Boston, in 2017. Hanna also writes children's books; *A Day in the Life of Nea* (2018) is a book about children's feelings and is available in English.

Danielle H. Maxonight, BFA, MSW, LCSW is a Certified Theraplay® Practitioner at Under Wing Therapeutic Services, PLLC, Asheville, North Carolina, USA. Danielle has worked in a variety of clinical settings, including a group home for foster youth near Detroit, two in-home therapy programs for rural Appalachian families in crisis, and a therapeutic boarding school for middle school girls from all over the world. Within these diverse settings, the prevalence of anxiety disorders cuts across geographical location, socio-economic status, race, age, gender and culture. Currently, she runs a private practice offering attachment-based therapy for (often anxious) school-aged children and their parents.

Nichole (Nicki) Melby, MMFT has completed Level 1 Theraplay® training and is a contributor to the chapter on Theraplay for children who are deaf or hard of hearing. Nicki has been deaf since the age of one and is fluent in American Sign Language. She has more than ten years of experience working in the field of adult mental health, including training in deaf pastoral studies. She did her internship with Alexis Greeves, where she learned about Theraplay. Nicki currently works at Volunteers of America and the Therapeutic Services Agency providing culturally affirmative and language-specific mental health services to children and their families.

Vivien Norris, DClinPsy, DipMusicTh is a chartered clinical psychologist and music therapist. She is also dually qualified as a Certified Theraplay® and Dyadic Developmental Psychotherapy Practitioner, Supervisor and Trainer. Vivien has worked as a clinical psychologist within the National Health Service in the UK for over 20 years and is now Clinical Director of The Family Place, an independent organization providing flexible therapeutic interventions for families. Vivien co-authored *Parenting with Theraplay* (2017) and *Theraplay: A Practical*

Guide for Practitioners (2020). She is the author of *By Your Side* (2019), a program focused specifically on the transition from fostering to adoption, including training, a children's book and foster carer, adopter and practitioner guides.

Fiona Peacock, MA, BACP is a senior accredited counselor and a Certified Theraplay® Practitioner, Supervisor and Trainer. Fiona is an affiliate lecturer in the Faculty of Education at the University of Cambridge and a therapist in private practice in the UK. She trained as a psychodynamic counselor and worked in Child and Adolescent Mental Health Services for over a decade as part of a specialist team for looked-after and adopted children. This experience led her to Theraplay training because she found traditional therapeutic techniques did not fully address the needs of this client group. Fiona is now in her final year of doctoral studies (EdD) researching Theraplay practice.

Saara Salo, PhD, a licensed clinical psychologist and parent-infant, family and emotion-focused couple's therapist, is a Certified Theraplay® Practitioner, Supervisor and Trainer. Saara is a Senior Affiliate at the University of Helsinki, and also has a private clinical practice. She has worked all her clinical career with pregnant couples, babies and families of young children mainly at the University Hospital of Helsinki. Saara has researched and published on the subjects of emotional availability during pregnancy (pre-EA), early parent-child intervention for depressed (Nurture and Play, NaP), substance-abusing mothers and the significance of a couple's relationship during the transition into parenthood. She is currently leading two large follow-up intervention studies.

Kay Schieffer, MA, MEd is a Certified Group Theraplay® Supervisor and Trainer, and the Executive Director of The Theraplay Institute in Evanston, Illinois, USA. Kay is a licensed special education teacher with over 25 years of experience in classrooms and behavioral health consultation. She is the developer of Sunshine Circles and author of the teacher's manual *Sunshine Circles: Nurture Your Classroom with Play* (second edition). Kay conducted two large-scale research investigations of the efficacy of Sunshine Circles as a social/emotional intervention in at-risk preschool classrooms in Iowa prior to taking her current position.

Lauren C. Smithee, MS, MFT, PhD candidate is a Foundational Theraplay® practitioner. She is a resident in marriage and family therapy and the recipient of the 2018 Theraplay Research Scholar Award. She became passionate about therapy with LGBTQ families due to her identification as a sexual minority woman in a same-gender marriage with a transgender woman. One of her areas of expertise is therapy with transgender people navigating couple and family relationships during transition. Lauren has sought numerous trainings to strengthen her skillset in intervention with LGBTQ families. She has published and presented her research related to LGBTQ families at local, regional and national conferences.

Chapter 1

An Overview of the Theraplay Model

*Sandra Lindaman, Rana Hong,
Danielle H. Maxonight and Fiona Peacock*

*Theraplay aims at causing simultaneous changes in the child's experience
of him or herself as more lovable and capable, of adults and especially their
parents as more safe and trustworthy and of the outside world as more
organized and joyful. At the same time it offers the parents a new view and
experience of their child. Seeing the well-being of one's own child enhances
one's own feelings of being worthy and is thus a potent organizer of mental
well-being for the parent also. And Theraplay gives a rare opportunity
to tend to the emotional hurts of the parents through not only mutual
mentalization and emotional attunement but through direct physical
co-regulation to diminish anxiety and enhance feeling good… Meanings
are supposedly the stuff of classical psychotherapy. But true meanings
are created when one experiences the sharing of one's bodily reality and
emotional reality in expanded, dyadic states of preverbal consciousness.
I know of no therapy geared more toward this than Theraplay.*

(Jukka Mäkelä, 2003, p.6)

Introduction

The Theraplay model is now over 50 years old and is growing and thriving.
The purpose of this book is to share with you how experienced Theraplay
practitioners have applied the model to specific populations and issues.
We are aware that we cannot convey this application information in a

first level of training, but also that it is what the trainee wants to know, because they work with those specific populations and issues. There are only so many topics that we can cover in one book; we plan to do another in the future with more applications, innovations and ways Theraplay is integrated with other treatment modalities. Readers who are not familiar with Theraplay may be inspired to seek training to learn a new approach to treatment.

Theraplay is a unique combination of active guidance by the practitioner, inclusion of the parent and child together, and face-to-face playful and caring interactions replicating experiences that are known to lead to secure attachment. One purpose of this chapter is to present an overview of Theraplay concepts and process as described in the third edition Theraplay text (Booth & Jernberg, 2010) so that chapter authors do not have to do so in each chapter—more room for implementation!

The other purpose of this chapter is to look at Theraplay through a slightly different lens, based on ten additional years of information from the world of neurobiology and psychotherapy. We understand more about how processes in Theraplay contribute to safety and arousal regulation. We describe how the dimensions contribute to attachment security. We now have a greater understanding of how a parent's own attachment history will influence the Theraplay process and how we work with that in parent-only sessions. We also understand more about how the Theraplay practitioner uses aspects of her/himself in this therapy where we are so present and active. Therefore, in this chapter we have offered thoughts on these four components of the Theraplay model: establishing safety and arousal regulation, enhancing caregiver-child attachment, working with the parents, and the practitioner's use of self.

Key points

Each author has been asked to identify key points about their topic. Our goal for this chapter is that readers, wishing to deepen their Theraplay practice, come to understand and internalize seven key points about Theraplay theory and process:

1. Theraplay is more than what happens in the treatment room between the practitioner, child and caregiver. Rather, Theraplay treatment consists of a particular sequence of events, including

interviews with the caregivers, observation of caregiver-child interaction, discussion and practice with the caregivers prior to treatment and during treatment, including the caregivers in weekly therapy sessions, and increasing the leadership role of the caregiver in sessions over time and homework.

2. The Theraplay dimensions of structure, engagement, nurture and challenge are the tools of Theraplay—all are equally important and are used together to create new experiences of safety, social engagement, co-regulation and attachment for caregivers and children.

3. Establishing client safety and arousal regulation is a foundation of the Theraplay process; the mutual social engagement and reciprocal play of Theraplay are beneficial factors in this process.

4. Enhancing caregiver-child attachment is achieved through strengthening the secure base through the dimensions by establishing the caregiver as a source of guidance and comfort, creating opportunities for affective synchrony and repair, and supporting exploration through experiences of pleasure and success.

5. Working directly with caregivers as they interact with their children in the treatment session and in separate practice, review and reflection meetings is a unique aspect of Theraplay treatment. In Theraplay, our work with the caregiver is just as important as our work with the child.

6. As Theraplay practitioners, we use aspects of ourselves, such as our own presence, social engagement, attunement, reflection and cultural humility, to create a good experience of being with another person for the caregiver, the child and the caregiver and child together.

7. The basic concepts of Theraplay's safety and attachment focus, dimensions and processes described in this chapter apply to dyadic parent-child work, Group Theraplay and Sunshine Circles.

The remainder of the chapter will describe these seven key concepts in Theraplay theory and practice.

The Theraplay assessment and treatment process

Theraplay is an effective dyadic psychotherapy consisting of a particular sequence of events:

1. Intake interviews with caregivers and gathering of relevant information about the family.

2. Direct observation of caregiver-child interactions via the Marschak Interaction Method (MIM).

3. Collaborative discussion of the MIM experience with the caregivers, and treatment planning employing the dimensions.

4. Caregiver-practitioner practice session, caregiver-child-practitioner weekly sessions.

5. Regular caregiver-practitioner reflective and practice sessions.

6. Termination and follow-up assessments and planning.

When Theraplay is used in settings where caregivers are not always present, such as in residential care or therapeutic education settings, extensive information about the child's behaviors in the setting will be considered in making a treatment plan.

The playful and caring activities employed in Theraplay sessions are designed to meet the treatment goals developed in the steps above. A practitioner who simply uses Theraplay activities without specific training in Theraplay and without following the above sequence, while pleasant and perhaps productive, is not doing Theraplay.

Note: Specific information about the assessment and planning process, including problem solving and addressing common practitioner questions, can be found in *Theraplay: The Practitioner's Guide* (Norris & Lender, 2020).

Theraplay dimensions of structure, engagement, nurture and challenge

Families come to Theraplay treatment because they are in distress. The presenting problem usually is the child's behavior. Caregivers often have tried parenting approaches based on rewards, time-outs, consequences and other treatments focused on helping the child talk about their feelings, calm themselves or solve problems. A caregiver who has been with the child since birth may or may not be aware that illness, separations, medical trauma, substance abuse, depression or exposure to domestic violence have had an effect on the developing child. A foster or adoptive caregiver may or may not know a great deal about their child's early experiences and the impact those experiences have on the child's way of relating to new caregivers. Caregivers usually have not considered how their responses to the child are influenced by the caregiver's own attachment history. The caregivers frequently are worn out and discouraged and feel ineffective.

The Theraplay assessment process begins to sort out what the child and caregiver's experiences have been and how current behaviors and patterns stem from these. We interview caregivers about the child's development and behaviors and the family history of life events while listening for attachment enhancing or thwarting themes and the caregiver's own history with respect to attachment. We observe child-caregiver interactions in the Marschak Interaction Method assessment, purposely giving tasks that call for aspects of security that we call the dimensions: structure, engagement, nurture and challenge. We hypothesize about what the child's and caregiver's internal working models (IWMs) are that guide their present behavior.

The behavior and relational patterns of many of our child clients suggest that they see themselves as unlovable or bad, others as uncaring or unable to help them, and the world as an uncomfortable place in which they don't fit. Children who have had severe neglect and abuse in their histories often have a more extreme view of self as not being worthy of protection and care, of others as overwhelming, and the world as a frightening place to be that they must control or collapse to diminish the threat. The caregiver's IWM will vary depending on the security of their own attachment history and subsequent life experiences; when they bring their child for treatment they often tell us that they feel ineffective, that their caregiving is negatively judged by others and that their caregiving world is difficult.

Theraplay treatment is the active creation of positive moments of interaction between caregiver and child that promote positive changes in IWMs and, therefore, in behaviors, feelings and thoughts. The intention is that through the structuring, engaging, nurturing and challenging aspects of the Theraplay experience, a new and more positive meaning of what it is like to be with another person may emerge.

Theraplay seeks to challenge the negative IWMs of child and caregiver, giving interactive and strong messages that child and caregiver are special and worthy, that the practitioner and caregiver are invested in hearing what the child is feeling and thinking and that the world is by and large safe and adults are responsible for keeping it that way.

The dimensions are building blocks of a secure base:

- *Structure.* The child experiences first the practitioner and then the caregiver as a person who can guide, organize and regulate his/her experiences. The caregiver develops leadership and regulating skills and uses them with growing confidence.

- *Engagement.* The child experiences first the practitioner and then the caregiver as a person who makes him/her feel present, seen, heard, felt and accepted through experiencing dyadic affective synchrony and repair. The caregiver experiences the power of reading and responding to the child's cues and connecting to their child with their face, eyes, voice, touch and movement.

- *Nurture.* The child experiences first the practitioner and then the caregiver as a person who can calm and soothe them and make them feel good physically and emotionally; the caregiver experiences success and satisfaction in meeting their child's needs.

- *Challenge.* The child experiences a strong sense of competence and mastery for his/her own abilities, while supported, celebrated and sometimes assisted first by the practitioner and then by the caregiver. The caregiver experiences success and competence in their ability to partner with and enjoy their child.

A Theraplay session of 30–40 minutes is composed of activities from all of the dimensions in a pattern, alternating more active and playful activities with less active and caring activities. This allows us to meet multiple needs for security in one session. It also gives us a way to give briefer experiences that may be difficult for the dyad, for instance quiet nurture, and then move to an interaction that is more comfortable for either the child or the caregiver, or both. Further information about how we apply these dimensions to enhance attachment is given later in this chapter.

Establishing safety and arousal regulation

This section considers ways that Theraplay promotes the *safety* of relationships. The child's physiological experience of safety and arousal state regulation is necessary for the development of affective regulation and attachment. Although safety clearly is a part of the attachment process, we have separated it here to focus on this detailed information that we have included in Theraplay thinking in the last five years.

Neuroscientist Cozolino notes:

> It is an unfortunate twist of evolutionary fate that the amygdala is mature before birth while the systems to inhibit it take years to develop. This leaves us vulnerable to overwhelming fear with little to no ability to protect ourselves. On the other hand, evolution has also provided us with caretakers who allow us to link into their developed cortex until ours is ready. The way they protect us from fear and modulate our anxiety becomes a model upon which our own brain develops. Thus, we use proximity to our parents as our key method of fear regulation… Our attachment schemas come to reflect the success or failure of how we and our parents navigate this process. (2010, p.253)

The infant's threat detection system includes cells in the brain stem responsible for mediating reactions to fight, flight or freeze responses that are triggered when the infant senses danger. These responses are part of the autonomic nervous system with its sympathetic (activating) and parasympathetic (calming) divisions (Siegel, 2012). The fear-processing amygdala in the limbic system is connected to the brain stem fight, flight or freeze defensive behaviors as well as to vigilance and stress hormone response systems (Baylin, 2018).

Bentsen and Hart explain the importance of these deep structures for all subsequent development:

> Feelings and expressions of pleasure and displeasure arise deep within subcortical structures, and vocal expressions and emotions, as well as the later emerging cognitive competencies that enable speech, depend on regulation in deep-seated structures in and around the brainstem and in the limbic system. The emergence of structures in the limbic system transforms self-regulation of arousal into emotions that motivate action…the development of the self-regulation capacity deep inside the basic subcortical structures shapes the organism's fundamental sense of trust and security. (2015, pp.3–4)

The caregiver's sensitivity in meeting the physical and emotional needs of the infant deactivates the stress response and self-defense systems. However, Baylin (2018) reminds us that, "through repeated exposure to threatening care, this brain system promotes chronic defensiveness" (p.37). Some children may not be able to receive the safety and sensitivity given by caregivers due to their neurological status, or due to overwhelming and/or isolating medical treatment. The chronic defensiveness also suppresses the development of higher brain regions and bilateral brain integration.

In Theraplay, we reduce defensive fear reactions and increase safety primarily through the dimensions of structure and nurture and the inclusion of and guidance to caregivers to give more reassuring messages to their children. Structure provided by an emotionally warm and regulated practitioner ensures order, predictability and regulation of the child's strong feelings. Repeated experience of nurture conveys the message that adults can be counted on to soothe and comfort the child. The parent work of direct guidance and reflection strengthens the sensitivity of their responses to the child. Upcoming attachment sections in this chapter will detail these areas. Polyvagal theory (PVT) (Porges, 2011, 2017, 2018) describes the neurophysiological foundations of safety and regulation. PVT suggests that Theraplay's engagement and type of play also are powerful tools to create safety for our clients.

Mental health practitioners working with adult survivors of trauma have incorporated PVT principles into various treatments in the last 20 years (Badenoch, 2018; Dana & Grant, 2018; Geller, 2018; Levine, 2018; Ogden, 2018; van der Kolk, 2018). More recently, those treating attachment-trauma problems have studied and incorporated PVT principles into treatment (Baylin, 2018; Baylin & Hughes, 2016; Kestly, 2016). It is not possible to describe PVT fully here; this section will focus on the aspects of the theory relevant to Theraplay, specifically the social engagement system, and the physiological states of play and intimacy. A great resource for learning more about PVT is *Clinical Applications of the Polyvagal Theory* (Porges & Dana, 2018), which includes a Theraplay chapter (Lindaman & Mäkelä, 2018).

Porges describes safety as a physiological state regulated by the autonomic nervous system (ANS) with sympathetic (SNS) and para-sympathetic (PNS) branches. The specific contribution of PVT (Porges, 2011, 2017, 2018) is the recognition that the vagus nerve has both ventral and dorsal vagal circuits; the circuits react in a hierarchy of response to threat. Porges created the term "neuroception" to describe mammals' unconscious, immediate evaluation of risk in the environment. Different patterns of response are associated with an evaluation of safety, danger or life threat.

A critical integration within mammals' nervous systems allows us to regulate each other through social behaviors, specifically facial expressions, vocalizations and gestures. PVT proposes that there is an integration of 1) the ventral vagal circuits that go from the brain to regulate the heart and bronchi and 2) the cranial nerves that supply the muscles for looking, facial expressions, vocalizing, listening, chewing, sucking, swallowing, breathing and gesturing with the head. This integration forms the social engagement system (SES). Through the SES, people give and receive signals of safety through their facial expressions, vocal prosody and head gestures. Porges says that these are the most potent safety signals. Essentially, when a person receives safety signals from the faces and voices of others, that person then neurocepts safety, their own SES is activated and they become social, get closer to others, and can be co-regulated by and develop trusting relationships with others.

If we are not experiencing a threat, our ventral vagus circuit (VVC) is activated. We can feel safe, connected and socially engaged, our emotions are tolerable and we can access our higher-level skills. Being in this socially engaged state inhibits the next set of defenses, if the internal/external stimuli are not too overwhelming, by containing the SNS and dorsal vagal circuit (DVC) in an optimal range. However, if we neurocept danger, the SNS mobilizes us to fight/flight behaviors. If that is not sufficient to deal with the danger, we experience life threat with activation of the DVC of the PNS leading to shut down/collapse/dissociation to escape the situation.

In addition to these three states of safety, danger and life threat, two additional states, play and intimacy, also are experienced as safe because they involve the VVC and safety cues from the SES. Polyvagal play is distinguished by reciprocal movement, proximity, touch and synchronous face-to-face interactions; the social engagement systems of the players (powered by the VVC) regulate the mobilization of their SNS and keep the players in the safe state (Porges, 2015). Giving and receiving nurture is another way to enter into and stay in a safe state. Intimacy, sometimes called "immobilization without fear" or "rest and digest," includes the prosocial use of the voice and face plus proximity and gentle contact allowing for intense down-regulation of arousal (powered by the DVC) while staying in connection (Porges, 2011).

Porges suggests that if we want to make the world safe for children we should work on "down-regulating defense and up-regulating social engagement" (2015, p.114). This fits with neuroscientist Baylin's description of a number of treatments focused on attachment-trauma problems (including Theraplay): "...all models work by helping quiet the chronically active defense system and promoting a brain awakening journey upward to prefrontal areas of brain" (2018, p.34). Baylin further explains:

> Using the three-state polyvagal model of the nervous system, we can think of trauma-focused therapy as a way for therapist and, with coaching, caregivers to use their social engagement system to co-regulate the child's states and help the child shift from the defensive nervous system to the social engagement system. Since the social engagement system is only accessible when the child experiences sufficient safety in the presence of an adult, the adult has to be adept at sending safety messages into the child's midbrain defense system to help the child make the desired shift from a defensive to an open state. (2018, p.42)

There is a strong coherence between three safe states described in PVT—social engagement, polyvagal play and intimacy—and three key aspects of Theraplay—engagement, play and nurture. Porges (2011) recommends ways to help children with attachment and behavior problems:

> We can alter the caregiving environment so that it will appear—and be—safer for children and less likely to evoke mobilization or immobilization responses. We also can intervene directly with children, exercising the neural regulation of brainstem structures, stimulating neural regulation of the SES, and encouraging positive social behaviour. (p.19)

Theraplay does precisely what Porges recommends; our manner of direct interpersonal engagement with clients, the very early nature of our play and care activities and our guidance of parents to engage in more sensitive and helpful interactions with their children are reasons for the often rapid and dramatic success we see in Theraplay.

PVT helps us understand that Theraplay contains many ways to enter, stay in, exercise and strengthen the safe state:

1. The way we warmly engage the child and caregiver via facial expression, vocal prosody, proximity and contact creates a sense of safety in the child/caregiver that allows them to become more socially engaged.

2. The way we initiate face-to-face, reciprocal and synchronous play with the child/caregiver allows them to experience a degree of sympathetic arousal without it spilling into fight/flight because it is mediated by the social engagement of the players—an experience of regulating each other.

3. The way we provide direct nurturing care is an experience of a safe degree of parasympathetic arousal which combines rest and digest states with social engagement and oxytocin from touch and contact.

4. The way we guide a sequence of play-care-play-care, all with social engagement, is an exercise of neural state regulation which enhances the flexibility of the SES and resilience.

Theraplay has always created opportunities for children and caregivers to experience something they have missed or don't have enough of: predictability, soothing, acceptance, attunement, connection, pleasure. Looking through the lens of PVT, we see that a Theraplay session takes place within the safe state where reciprocal social engagement is possible. This safe state experience is often unfamiliar and hard for the child and caregiver to create on their own.

As we assess dyads, we need to pay attention to what degree of social engagement or defensiveness the child and caregiver show through their faces, voices, proximity, contact and level of arousal. Fortunately, we have an excellent tool in the Marschak Interaction Method to observe these signs and assess such patterns. We can factor this into our discussions with parents and treatment planning. Then the child-caregiver sessions create new ways of entering the safe state through the leadership of the practitioner, the attraction of play and the comfort of sensitively given nurture. Participating in social engagement successfully increases the sense of safety and tolerance for emotions and stimulation. We provide periods of up-regulating interactive play, followed by periods of down-regulating nurturing care, in a play-care-play-care sequence throughout the session. When Theraplay is viewed through a polyvagal lens, the entire

Theraplay process can be seen as an exercise of neural regulation leading to enhanced safety and reduced defensiveness.

Enhancing caregiver-child attachment

Only after the careful preparation of the assessment protocol do we enter parent-child play sessions, with the goal of giving new experiences designed to counter unhelpful IWMs. Practitioner-guided play, care and reflection are the vehicles through which we offer a special type of presence to families. Our presence, more than any specific protocol or Theraplay activity, will promote the dyad's growing security. What we have playfully nicknamed "the Theraplay way" could also be called, less memorably, "the way of secure caregivers." So what exactly is "the Theraplay way"? Here are four attachment-promoting processes we set into motion:

1. Intentional, sensitive leadership.

2. Opportunities for the child to turn to and receive comfort from the caregiver.

3. Affective synchrony and interactive repair.

4. Experiences of exploration, pleasure and joint success.

Attachment processes will be described briefly and illustrated through the Theraplay process and treatment examples.

Intentional, sensitive leadership

Theraplay provides a felt experience of the caregiver as a friendly, calm and confident guide. Secure caregivers are "bigger, stronger, wiser, and kind"; this helps the child feel protected and self-assured, able to relax, explore, take risks and reach their full potential (Bowlby, 1969, 1988; Powell *et al.*, 2014). The caregiver embodies "confident presence" in a way that is "clear, expressed unobtrusively, and available when needed—in a way, hidden in plain sight" (Powell *et al.*, 2014, p.143). In Theraplay, we provide just this type of relating. We plan and guide sessions based on our evolving theory of the dyad's needs. We set clear limits. We use directives, proximity, touch and playfulness to create structure. We do this to give a new experience to dyads where structure may have been non-existent, inconsistent, confusing, harsh or at a too mature level for the child.

However, the core of structure is not in the specifics of what we say or do, but in how we say and do it. We embody emotional warmth, self-assuredness and trustworthiness, and we use our tone of voice, body language and facial expressions to communicate this non-verbally. For example, we might decide to move on from an activity a child is rejecting by saying, "Let's try something new!" This simple statement could be said in an exasperated, defeated tone that collapses the structure, relinquishing our responsibility to the child and undermining security; however, the Theraplay practitioner says it in a playful, confident, firm way that fully provides structure and indicates that something else good is coming.

Another aspect of structure is the physical setting and sequence of a Theraplay session. Practitioner, child and caregiver usually sit on the floor together on a mat, carpet or blanket, supported with pillows for their comfort and close enough that the participants can make contact. This is not always possible due to the individual's physical limitations or doing Theraplay in someone's home, but there is still an intention to create a comfortable, informal play space, perhaps with a bean-bag chair or small rug the practitioner brings with them. Simple play materials are kept in a bag and activities are presented one at a time. By participating in this process, the child is relieved of the burden of figuring out what to do next or how to keep themselves safe. Each session has the same basic structure, and activities have clear beginnings and endings. A typical sequence would be:

1. The practitioner, caregiver and child enter the treatment space in a pleasant, connected way (e.g., holding hands and taking big steps to pillows on the floor).

2. The therapist sits across from the child and caregiver, notices their special personal features and, with the caregiver's help, attends to any "hurts" the child may have.

3. Up-regulating activity (e.g., popping bubbles with fingers, knees, elbows).

4. Down-regulating, caring activity (e.g., making powder handprints).

5. Up-regulating activity (e.g., jumping off a stack of pillows into the caregiver's arms).

6. Additional sequences of up- and down-regulating based on the child's window of affect tolerance.

7. Down-regulating, soothing activity (e.g., sharing a food treat, drink, song).

8. Exit with the caregiver and child connected (e.g., piggy-back ride to door).

The practitioner leads this process by choosing and pacing activities at therapeutically appropriate levels of arousal. The practitioner briefly explains one activity at a time while leading the child through the activity. If a child is reluctant to interact, the practitioner demonstrates on themselves or with the parent. The practitioner decides when and how much to ask the caregiver to lead activities. When activities become familiar, explanations are not necessary and the practitioner introduces small variations to maintain interest; for instance, if the child has been popping bubbles blown by the practitioner, the practitioner could practice and then call out different ways to pop the bubble, such as "Clap them… Grab them… Poke them."

If a child is very fast moving and impulsive, we often use signals to help them wait for a cue word or eye blink to take their turn. Alternatively, if the child is very rigid and timid, we loosen the structure and encourage any initiatives of the child, for instance making a child's small finger wiggle into a way to push a cotton ball off a pillow or towards the practitioner.

The practitioner leads the child through a series of playful activities that provide an organized, regulated interpersonal experience.

 The practitioner sets up an activity with larger and then smaller movements and louder and quieter voices for an easily dysregulated child. The child, father and practitioner all hold the edges of a blanket between them. The practitioner places a pillow in the center of the blanket and tells the group they will toss it up on the count of three. It goes fairly high and all celebrate noisily. Then, in a calmer and quieter voice, the practitioner says, "Now let's do it lower next time so it's just a little toss." The child, reacting to the practitioner's calmer tone of voice, looks at her intently. The next toss is lower and the practitioner observes, "It does go lower; oh look, we're good at that." Next, they do it "really high" and it gets stuck in the ceiling fan! A moment of surprise for all; the child grabs the pillow and begins to run away with it. The practitioner gets him back by suggesting that they do a bigger pillow and then two pillows at once. Suddenly the child says "A little lower" in the same tone used by the practitioner earlier. They do it as the child suggested and he smiles. The practitioner feels that this sequence is complete and switches to an activity requiring a more coordinated action, passing a balloon from person to person around the blanket. This is accomplished successfully. Then the child is directed to sit in the blanket so the adults can swing him while the adults sing to him. The child eagerly accepts this.

Another positive message is that there are no hurts in a Theraplay session. Practitioners introduce this proactively, for instance saying, "I'm going to blow these bubbles toward you but I'm going to take care that they don't get in your eyes. It's my job to be sure that there are no hurts in here." Another is that the practitioner takes responsibility for failures, for instance saying, "Wow, I forgot how hard it could be to punch through four sheets of newspaper. I forgot to try three first."

The predictability of the session sequence itself can be reassuring to children who have experienced a great deal of chaos.

 In the sixth month of Theraplay treatment, a very dysregulated child with a history of severe abuse and neglect enters a session yelling about his terrible day and resisting contact. Knowing that he could easily escalate to aggression if approached, the practitioner stays with the child, acknowledges what a bad day it has been, and allows the child to calm down in the nest of pillows on the floor. After many minutes, the child begins to calm down; he talks about what he has seen out of the window and reflects about positive interactions with the practitioner in past sessions. Suddenly the child says, in a curious and expectant tone of voice, "So, what do we got today...can I look in the bag?" Then the practitioner engages the boy and his father in a series of nurturing and structuring activities to communicate that the child is accepted and liked despite his explosion and that the child is capable of participating in positive, regulated interactions with others.

We involve the caregivers in the interaction in a variety of ways depending on their comfort and the child's acceptance of the parent as a leader. First, they sit beside their child and see how the practitioner interacts with the child. Gradually they take turns with the child in activities. Even at a point when a caregiver does several activities with their child in a row, the practitioner is right there, assisting and supporting the dyad. There is more information about parent participation later in this chapter (see Working with caregivers).

When a child feels that their caregiver sensitively guides and regulates them, they can comfortably turn to the caregiver to relieve their physical and emotional distress. Next, we will discuss these very early caregiver-child interactions and how we offer reparative experiences through the dimension of nurture.

Creating opportunities for the child to turn to the caregiver to receive comfort

Schore (2009) tells us:

> Secure attachment depends on the mother's sensitive psychobiological attunement to the infant's dynamically shifting internal states of arousal. Through visual-facial, auditory-prosodic, and tactile-gestural communication, caregiver and infant learn the rhythmic structure of the other and modify their behavior to fit that structure, thereby co-creating a specifically fitted interaction. (pp.116–117)

In the first two months of the infant's life the caregiver's role is to give life-preserving and growth-facilitating physical and emotional care. Schore and Marks-Tarlow (2018) point out that Winnicott (1963) referred to this interaction as "quiet love" "seen in the moments when the mother holds and handles (soothes, comforts and caresses) the infant" (p.67). The mother's close attention to and following of the infant attunes her to the infant's physical and emotional needs. The way the caregiver attends to the child's signals, figures out what they mean for the child and responds contingently is critical. In these first few months of life, quiet love makes it possible for the distress of a wet, cold, hungry or in some way uncomfortable infant to be transformed to comfort and relief. In terms of what is happening in the infant's body and brain, the distress, which is felt as strong, unpleasant sympathetic activation of the autonomic nervous system, is down-regulated to a positive, calming, pleasant parasympathetic state; "both mother and baby are primarily engaged at the subcortical level of amygdala, mediating basic emotions" (ibid, p.71).

Theraplay provides direct care experiences between the caregiver and child in the session; additionally, the practitioner maintains a caring, attentive mindset towards the caregiver and child at all times. We do this to replicate the critical message that a baby receives through body contact with the caregiver—that someone can calm and soothe the child and make them feel good physically and emotionally.

 A three-year-old child in foster care (who we will call Jenny) is described as extremely independent and "doesn't fuss or argue but does whatever she wants to." She sometimes takes food, hides under a bed and does not respond to the calls of people looking for her. Jenny had been removed from her biological parent at birth due to her drug exposure and a serious illness requiring nine months of hospitalization in a long-term pediatric ward. When placed with the foster carer, she insisted on holding her own bottle and "toilet trained herself" quite early. The foster carer said that Jenny's self-sufficiency made her easy to care for, but she worried about her future. In a Theraplay session, the practitioner paints lotion on the child's hand and presses it down on a sheet of dark paper to make a hand print. She then rubs the lotion gently into Jenny's hand, singing "Oh lotion, oh lotion on Jenny's hand, it feels so good, it feels so grand." Jenny cocks her head and stares at the practitioner in amazement as if the practitioner is speaking an unknown but interesting language. In the next session, the foster mom makes a print of Jenny's feet, rubs in the lotion and sings the song and then holds a juice box while Jenny takes sips from it. When Mom gives Jenny a cookie, the practitioner gives a cookie to Mom so that they can crunch them at the same time. After only a few of these sessions, Jenny comes to Mom for help at home and does not hide from others. During a check-up phone call, the foster mom tells the practitioner, "She calls you the 'Oh Lotion Lady.'"

The care or nurture aspects of Theraplay are unique in child therapy: singing, rocking, feeding, paying attention to the body, caring for hurts. Each session contains several caring activities, at the beginning and ending of sessions and often in the middle. As noted in the safety section, such caring activities using touch paired with safety cues of warm facial expressions and prosodic voice from the social engagement systems of the practitioner and caregiver can further enhance the child's neuroception of safety and the strength and flexibility of the child's social engagement system. Mäkelä in Bentzen and Hart (2015) describes the benefit of "steady, rhythmic deep touch that calms the child down by sending signals to deep-seated centers in the brain that increase oxytocin levels and, thus, the feeling of well being in another person's company" (p.173). Theraplay's nurture:

> is not intended to encourage regression, but rather to answer the questions that went unanswered for far too long during child's first year of life: "Is someone taking full responsibility for looking after me, making sure my body feels good; good enough to make living worthwhile?" (Mäkelä in Bentzen & Hart, 2015, pp.79–80)

Sometimes we have the opportunity to work with an infant and caregiver in Theraplay (see Chapter 3), but the majority of our clients are well beyond infancy and have often suffered a lack of safety and basic trust, and the consequences of living for years without them. The nurture that is always offered in a Theraplay session tells the child that their need for comfort:

- won't be dismissed as unnecessary, babyish, attention seeking or manipulative
- is not dependent on their good behavior
- can feel safe and good, even if touch and closeness were frightening in the past
- can be met by their caregiver instead of always taking care of themselves
- does not mean they have to take care of their caregiver.

As in the example above, the practitioner usually begins the direct nurture of the child and also offers indirect or direct nurture to the caregiver as appropriate. However, the goal of Theraplay is that the caregiver should be the nurture giver as soon as possible. The caregiver may not have had positive experiences of nurture themselves. They may tell us that caregiving is babying or spoiling, creates dependency or rewards bad behavior, is unimportant or contrary to their desire to "toughen up" their child. They may tell us they are uncomfortable with nurture. In separate parent-only meetings, we discuss how the caregiver came to have these beliefs, review the session video to think about the effect of nurture on the child, and practice with the parent. This process is described later in this chapter (Working with caregivers).

In contrast to the dimensions of structure, engagement or challenge, nurture is given directly, without playing, unless the child or caregiver have difficulty accepting or giving care; in that case, more playful methods can be tried in response to the client's unfamiliarity or reluctance, for instance a child who will not allow himself to be fed may participate in a taste test of different flavored chips handed to him one at a time while the practitioner and caregiver try to guess his favorite from his facial expression. We always have something to eat and drink available. We never insist on accepting touch or food. We look for alternate, less intense ways to convey care—for example, fanning the child's hands after she punches a newspaper, or wiping off their hands after poking bubbles— and wait for the child to become more comfortable.

We learn about the child and caregiver's experiences with nurture before we nurture them. Prior to the first Theraplay session we have information about how the dyad responds to proximity, touch and care because we have gathered details about the caregiver-child early life experiences, we have observed the caregiver and child in the MIM in dyadic nurturing activities and we have practiced nurturing activities with the caregiver and reflected about how the caregiver felt and the child might respond to nurture prior to the child session. We realize that some children and caregivers may have experienced abusive touch; therefore we go slowly and monitor the client's reactions to contact carefully. With the child and caregiver in session we acknowledge both verbally and non-verbally any discomfort that we suspect, and change what we are doing. However, as Mäkelä in Bentzsen and Hart (2015) points out, "close physical contact and touch are never questioned *per se*, as they are crucial aspects of both engagement and nurturing" (p.79), and also "to avoid using touch means abandoning the child to him/herself in a tough world, where the only reliable source of pleasure and joy is to be found individually, in isolation, which is likely to feed addiction issues" (p.173).

Humans need safety and co-regulation through the lifespan to feel good and reach their highest potential. The patterns of safety and regulation established through "quiet love" in the early months continue throughout childhood in more mature forms and are offered as a form of safe haven when a child is stressed. In Theraplay sessions, we establish soothing rituals of physical care and attention and continue to use them in each session throughout treatment.

In the next stage of infant development, more elaborate interactions focused on affective attunement, synchrony and repair are possible.

Affective synchrony and interactive repair

Schore (2009) describes:

> In play episodes of affective synchrony, the pair experiences a condition of resonance, and, in such, an amplification of vitality affects and a positive state occurs. In moments of interactive repair, the "good enough" caregiver who has misattuned can regulate the infant's negative state by accurately reattuning in a timely manner. The regulatory processes of affective synchrony that creates positive arousal and interactive repair that modulates negative arousal are the fundamental building blocks of attachment and its associated emotion. (p.117)

Theraplay's dimension of engagement provides attuned responsiveness during simple reciprocal play through which the child experiences themselves as being seen and felt as a distinct and valued individual and comes to enjoy interpersonal contact. These playful interactions create many opportunities for new experiences of affective synchrony and repair of the ingrained negative effects of previous unrepaired misattunements.

 A seven-year-old child who has been very neglected from birth to two years is frequently explosive and often disengaged from her caregivers. In her fourth Theraplay session, she sits in her adoptive father's lap and faces her adoptive mom. The practitioner suggests that mom and daughter fill their cheeks with air, put their hands to their faces, and softly pop their own cheeks at the same time. Mom is directed to watch her child closely and time her pop just at the moment the child pops. They pop and then laugh in delight at their shared experience. They repeat this, sometimes with perfect coordination and sometimes with misses, but they continue to adjust, laugh and smile. The caregivers later reflect that their daughter probably has never experienced the pleasure of back and forth "baby games" and the knowledge that adults want to play like this with her.

This type of attuned play is a feature of a second stage of mother-infant interaction that emerges in the second to third months of life once the autonomic and central nervous systems are more mature. Schore and Marks-Tarlow (2018) describe the infant as better able to focus interpersonally, so the mother starts to play "in intimate and affectionate ways that express reciprocal and intense engagement" (p.72). Winnicott refers to this as "excited love" when the mother helps the child transition from a calm, alert state into a regulated high-arousal state in which the sympathetic nervous system is activated and the infant experiences expanding joy and excitement, akin to Fromm's (1956) "love of life." The dyad is now interacting at the level of the limbic system. The mother and child participate in "protoconversations" by exchanging and maintaining sequences of head and body movements, hand gestures, facial expressions and vocalizations in which they influence each other. Trevarthen and Aitken (2001) use the term primary intersubjectivity to describe this shared state of attention, feelings and intentions. There is a third stage of these affective exchanges at 10–12 months associated with the beginning of a period of growth in the infant's neocortical, emotion-regulating area of the orbitofrontal cortex. This involves stretching affect tolerance by even stronger expressions of emotional arousal and experiencing more novelty (Schore & Marks-Tarlow, 2018).

We often see children who have experienced significant neglect and abuse; they have not experienced quiet love or excited love and indeed do not seem to have a "love of life" but rather live in distress and hyperarousal or, sometimes, collapse. Because their early experiences did not include soothing and feelings of safety, nor basic affective synchrony and repair, their path to the third level of neocortical development is impeded. Theraplay gives these children an experience of a new kind of relationship in place of inattention to and/or misreading of the child's cues, or caregivers who responded to their own needs rather than the child's. In this new kind of relationship, the intersubjective experience of affect synchrony can feel safe and rewarding.

Dissanayake (2001) explains that the experience of affective synchrony with the mother sends "positive affiliative messages about intentions and feelings, such as: You interest me, I like you, I am like you, I like to be with you, You please me, I want to please you, You delight me, I want to communicate with you, I want you to be like me" (p.91). These are the same messages that our engaging Theraplay interactions convey.

It is even possible to convey these important messages to older children.

 A 16-year-old boy enters residential care after living on the street for several years. His early life had been full of trauma and chaos. He attends treatment with a Theraplay practitioner and a staff member from his unit as his "primary carer" in the facility. In the first activity, he skillfully pokes and chops through many sheets of newspaper held tautly in front of him by his carer. He seems pleased by the amazed reactions of the practitioner and carer. Then the youth and carer sit face to face on a small couch, their knees almost touching and their faces about 36 inches apart. The practitioner has them cup their outstretched hands and blow a feather back and forth between them; as they do this they bob and weave closer and farther away from each other and also make effortful and breathy sounds. The practitioner suggests that they copy each other's sounds and they produce a series of growls, squeaks and raspberries that match the other in pitch and intensity; although not asked, they also copy each other's facial expressions and body movements. The practitioner gives it a bit more structure by having them repeat a word or short phrase in the same way; again, loud, soft, squeaky, rumbling sounds are matched. The youth prolongs an "OOOOO" in a musical way and the carer pays close attention and imitates it. Then they prolong the sound and match each other precisely as they raise and lower the pitch for seconds at a time. They laugh at the sound and the shared experience; the youth reaches out to the face of the carer; the carer smiles and squeezes his hand.

As we can see in the example above, Theraplay has specific techniques for promoting synchrony:

- Close positioning and face-to-face interactions so that the child has a clear impression of our face, voice and gestures and we are in the best position to see and respond to small initiatives from the child.

- Focus on the players, not object/toy use; even if an item is used with older children, it is to facilitate interpersonal interaction, not to focus on the item.

- Synchronous movements, usually with body contact, for example clapping games, hand stacks, row your boat.

- Preverbal level of interaction rather than word based.

- Matching of faces, voices, movements, for example copying each other's faces, voice tone, movements.

- Focus on the reaction of the other, and on adjustments, for example the child and caregiver "decorate" each other with stickers, feathers, crepe paper strips.

- Deeply interpersonal experiences that are also multisensory, involving vision, hearing, touch, movement, proprioception, smell and taste.

Tronick and Beeghly (2011) remind us that the lovely coordinated dance of shared positive affect between caregiver and infant is achieved only about 20–30 percent of the time—the rest is "messy": "it moves from matching (coordinated, synchronous) states of shared meanings and intentionality to mismatched (miscoordinated, dyssynchronous) states and back to matching intentional states via an active, jointly carried out reparatory process" and that "periods of dyadic matching are associated with the infant's positive affect and engagement, whereas dyadic mismatches are associated with infant's negative affect and dysregulation" (p.112). They propose that the dyad's ability or lack of ability to repair gives critical messages to the infant. Repair leads to implicit relational knowing that "we can repair mismatches"; this knowledge leads to a "sense of trust and eventually to a secure attachment relationship with that person" (p.113). Additionally, the feeling of success contributes to a beginning sense of mastery, a positive mood and a sense of well-being which allow the child to approach new, unknown situations with a positive feeling. Alternatively, a failure to repair mismatches, with the following dysregulation and negative affect, leads to a sense for the child that they cannot get help controlling their feelings and that they are stuck in the bad feeling. Tronick and Beeghly state, "This sense of failure may lead to an insecure attachment relationship with that person and may undermine the infant's sense of trust in others" (2011, p.113).

Children who have had insufficient affective synchrony and many failed repairs often do not give strong signals of discomfort due to a lack of trust in others. If they do give a signal, some caregivers ignore, minimize or try to talk the child out of a negative feeling. So, the Theraplay practitioner watches for the child's non-verbal messages of uncertainty or concern in order to demonstrate a new kind of response. For example, when the practitioner rubs lotion on the child's hand and the child pulls away with a look of disgust and shakes her hands in wordless distress, we attune to her affect, match our face with the child's, and state, "Yuck! Lotion! You're letting me know you don't like the feeling of that! Let me wipe that lotion away for you." In video review and discussion with the caregiver, we point out the child's relief and acceptance of more connection that generally follows the acknowledgment of "something is wrong."

We can even set up "practice" for the caregiver to watch for and respond to signals.

 The adoptive parents of a six-year-old son, who experienced severe neglect from birth to age four, tell us that he often has negative facial expressions which they cannot figure out; they generally interpret them as boredom. In a Theraplay session, the child sits with his bare foot outstretched to his adoptive dad. The practitioner asks Dad to wiggle each toe as he says "This little piggy likes…" and complete the phrase with a favorite food of the child. Dad is instructed to watch the child's face carefully to see if he agrees with him or not. The child lights up, smiling and chuckling as Dad names his favorites. When Dad says "waffles" there is a moment of tension when the child frowns and says in a whining tone, "I don't like waffles." The practitioner says, "Dad, he let us know, didn't he? I'll bet you can think of another." Dad fills in another word, the child nods and smiles, and the engagement continues.

Rather than ask a child how they are feeling, Theraplay practitioners look for non-verbal cues. We acknowledge and name the feelings a child reveals non-verbally and verbally, just as sensitive caregivers do. Some children have had very little experience with this acknowledgment and some caregivers skip the step and expect the child to take responsibility for the telling. Powell *et al.* (2014) suggest, "It is through the repeated process of parents helping their children recognize, name, assign meaning to, and deal with internal experiences that children become competent in managing feelings both by themselves and in relationship" (p.31). This ability is central to security.

A mother of an eight-year-old child adopted four years ago tells us that her child never tells her how she feels. We can see that the child is quiet and has a flat affect. In the MIM feedback we share our hypothesis that the child has not had enough "mind-reading" in her early life to now verbalize her feelings and would benefit from our reading her non-verbal cues. Mom says that the child doesn't give those either. So, in session we look for those non-verbal signs and help the parent respond to them instead of waiting for words. We may set up an activity of the child punching through a sheet of newspaper held tautly by the practitioner and Mom; when the child appears engaged and happy to have punched through one and then two sheets of paper, we ask Mom to look at her facial expression and decide if it means they should do more. Mom says "Yes!" and the child says "Yay" and punches again. In another activity of putting lotion on a child's freckles, she eagerly shows us a hurt on her knee and Mom is given lotion to put around it. When Mom encourages the child to show a bruise on her back, the child looks self-conscious and refuses. Mom insists briefly, but we say aloud that it looks as if the child is not comfortable with showing us, but certainly Mom can check at home and give it special attention. Mom says she thinks it was okay, but sees that the child didn't feel that. The practitioner reviews what just happened by copying the child's refusal movement and saying, "You let us know you didn't want to show us— that's what Mom wants to know." Mom says in a very warm voice, "You can show me anything you want." When she reaches out and rubs the child's foot, the child smiles and relaxes.

Having considered how Theraplay provides new experiences of being cared for by a bigger, stronger, wiser adult who is able to keep the child safe and soothed, delighted in and understood, we now turn to celebrate the child's exploration and success.

Experiences of exploration, pleasure and success
Bowlby (1988) described:

> the provision by both parents of a secure base from which a child or an adolescent can make sorties into the outside world and to which he can return knowing for sure that he will be welcomed when he gets there,

nourished physically and emotionally, comforted if distressed, reassured if frightened. (p.11)

The Theraplay dimension of challenge can be seen as a practice of "sorties into the outside world" in which the child can experience strong feelings of competence and mastery for their own abilities while being cheered on, assisted as needed and celebrated by the practitioner and caregiver. The child and caregiver together manage pleasure and success as well as effort, frustration and higher levels of arousal.

Challenge celebrates the age and interest of the child, to see him as a child ready to explore. Distinct from nurturing activities which meet the child's younger needs, these challenge activities feel more age appropriate and satisfy the child's desire to move and to be seen as the age that he or she is. A Theraplay colleague describes the dimension of challenge as "showing the child who he is" (Miwa Takai, personal communication, 2015).

 A six-year-old boy with past medical trauma and very withdrawn behavior has become much more engaged and accepting of nurture through the Theraplay sessions. Now he is ready to take a risk: the practitioner puts a sturdy pillow on the floor and has the caregiver stand on one side of it and the child on the other. Mom gives a cue for the child to jump up on the pillow with both feet and he succeeds with a grin. Pillows are added to the stack, and with each jump up, the child becomes taller and better balanced; the adults noisily celebrate the child's success. When four pillows are stacked and jumped on successfully, the child says with delight and amazement, "I can't believe I'm doing this!"

Challenge activities are not just a child accomplishing something with the caregivers watching, but also an opportunity to feel the pleasure and partnership in the child-caregiver experience. Many of our clients have had so many experiences of feeling incompetent with their peers and within their family that their self-esteem suffers. We carefully choose challenges that we believe are doable; if the child struggles, we take responsibility and find a way for the basic activity to be more successful. Thus, we ensure success for the child. We also help the caregiver to adjust their expectations to be developmentally on target, to deal with their own competitiveness, and to focus on fun rather than rules and sportsmanship.

We set up a new flow of experiences between the child and caregivers with clear achievable activities, assistance as needed, and immediate and positive feedback.

To figure out what is doable, practitioners may rehearse a simple version of a challenge to give a feeling of success; if that is successful, more challenge can be added.

 Mom, Dad, child and practitioner sit in a circle and hold the edges of a large square scarf between them. They raise it up to their faces and all look and smile at each other. The practitioner puts a feather on the scarf, leans over and blows it down the side of the scarf to Mom, Mom blows it to the child, the child to Dad, and it goes around the circle. The family enjoys the activity and successfully gets the feather around the scarf three times. The practitioner proposes something even "more fun." The family members stand and each is given a small throw pillow. Dad puts a feather on his pillow and blows it over to his child. She catches it on her pillow, sometimes having to dive for it. This is much harder and they miss the feather more than they catch it. The mother begins to correct the child and the child wilts. The practitioner says, "Wait a minute, I see what I did wrong!" She replaces the small pillows with bigger ones. Now they catch them and celebrate.

We also use challenge to help a child channel some escalating, negative physical actions (e.g., running around the room or throwing objects) into a more focused, controlled and positive action, such as slowing the running down so that he can still hold a feather on his palm and not lose it while he moves. Caregivers are troubled and usually feel helpless when they see their child's behavior escalate; they benefit from seeing and participating in concrete ways to redirect and re-engage the child.

As we know, increasing the security of the child's attachment to the caregiver has critical and life-long benefits. Siegel (2012) describes secure relationships as having many positive outcomes for children, including "the ability to balance one's emotions, to reduce fear, to be attuned to others, to have insight and self-understanding, to have empathic understanding of others, and to have well developed moral reasoning" (pp.20–5 & 206). Wallin (2007) describes secure attachment as related to "substantially greater self-esteem, emotional health and ego resilience, positive affect, initiative, social competence, and concentration in play" (p.23). Theraplay's focus on dyadic guiding, protecting, caring, attuning, repairing, playing and celebrating creates a new meaning of togetherness for the child and caregiver, gives the caregiver new tools and a deeper understanding of the child, and supports the child's healthy development.

We turn now to discuss our work with parents in greater detail.

Working with caregivers

Working directly with caregivers is a unique aspect of Theraplay treatment. We see the "client" as the caregiver-child relationship and caregivers as powerful, insightful allies with much to offer the change process. Theraplay practitioners strive to understand caregivers and to demonstrate compassion for them. We do this in a number of ways, including exploring the caregiver's own childhood experiences (see Chapter 2), supporting new meaning-making around the presenting problem, shoring up the caregiver in play sessions, and celebrating the caregiver's growth process via review of video clips.

Most caregivers who seek treatment for their children are experiencing shame, anxiety, frustration and confusion in their day-to-day caregiving role. Although on the surface a caregiver may blame their child or seem numbly resigned, beneath these defense mechanisms, the caregiver's narrative is usually one of failure, of "being a bad caregiver." Our first goal is to support a reappraisal process that allows the caregiver to move out of shame and develop a coherent, compassionate story for the presenting concerns (Baylin, 2017). This typically means connecting the current relational strife to a child's diagnosis with hereditary risk factors; family stress in key phases of a child's development due to death, illness, the birth of a sibling, a move, or loss of income; a caregiver's difficulty with certain aspects of caregiving because of their own difficult upbringing or diagnosis; and/or a mismatch in temperament, energy level or sensory needs between caregiver and child. When relevant, we draw on Baylin and Hughes' (2016) concept of "blocked care" to help a caregiver know that painful biological processes underlie their difficulty in freely feeling and conveying affection towards their traumatized child. By sharing many new possibilities, we offer a more realistic, redeeming theory for the dyad's troubles. This builds hope.

Whenever possible, we emphasize caregivers' strengths. We find ways to compliment them in front of their children as we play. For example, when a caregiver rubs lotion on their child's dry hands, the practitioner might say, "Your mom knows just how to make you feel better!" In caregiver-only review sessions, we select positive and successful moments to shore up the caregiver's fragile confidence. With difficult segments of video, we empathize with the caregiver's position, wonder with the caregiver about their feelings in the particular clip, and compassionately hold and organize their distress. The caregiver's needs—not the child's—are most important to us in these moments.

Offering the four dimensions to caregivers

In Theraplay, we assume a parallel process between the caregiver's relationship with their child and the practitioner's relationship with that caregiver. We know that all caregivers have a history of being parented imperfectly. It is too difficult for a caregiver to give their child relational "gifts" that they themselves never received. To resolve this issue, we must provide caregivers with the same relational qualities we believe their child will benefit from: nurture, engagement, structure and challenge.

Our "gift-giving" happens both directly, through our experiential practice of Theraplay activities with caregivers, and less concretely, through our general way of being with them. Offering hot tea, cough drops or an adjustment on the thermostat are simple, tangible ways to *nurture* caregivers. We also nurture caregivers with warm eye contact and unconditional positive regard. We *engage* caregivers by co-regulating their affect, mirroring their body language, facial expression and voice tone and suggesting words for their complex feelings. We create "now moments"—surprise and delight—by laughing with caregivers and celebrating with them. Rarely has a caregiver been stoic in the face of a big high five to congratulate a baby step. Our clear boundaries and predictable responses create *structure*. Some caregivers benefit from summary handouts, for example a PDF explaining the stages of Theraplay or their role in treatment. This supplies a clear framework and a sense of security. Lastly, we *challenge* caregivers to embody many new caregiving skills, scaffolding their development throughout the entire Theraplay journey.

Building caregivers' reflective functioning

Reflective functioning is referred to at different times as theory of mind (Premack & Woodruff, 1978), reflective function (Fonagy, Steele & Steele, 1991), mindsight (Siegel, 1999), mind-mindedness (Meins *et al.*, 2002) or mentalization (Fonagy *et al.*, 2002). At its core, reflective functioning is the "capacity to perceive and understand oneself and others in terms of psychological states that include feelings, beliefs, intentions and desires" (Powell *et al.*, 2014, p.35). Since we can never truly know the mind of another person, reflective functioning is a process of making careful observations, guessing and being open to "getting it wrong." Research shows that parental reflective functioning can predict parent-child relational outcomes, with stronger reflective functioning leading to relationships with more parental involvement, communication, satisfaction, limit setting and support (Rostad & Whitaker, 2016).

We build reflective functioning in Theraplay treatment in a variety of ways, including a review of videotaped sessions. The practitioner says to a caregiver, "Your child starts tapping his foot right here. I wonder if he is feeling frustrated or anxious about what I just said? Or maybe he is really excited and ready for me to move on? I'm not so sure…" We communicate with uncertainty and offer many possibilities in order to model and promote reflective functioning. Our lack of certainty helps caregivers loosen their (often unhelpful) fixed notions about their child's motives.

To encourage caregivers' engagement in this process, we show short segments of video and ask questions such as:

- Putting yourself back in that moment, what were you feeling?

- What do you imagine your child might be experiencing here?

- What do you guess your child really needed from me?

- What do you think your child might be trying to tell us when he jumps around excitedly, clears his throat like that, hides under the blanket, pushes my hand away?

Robust reflective functioning allows caregivers to develop an open and compassionate state of mind about their child's "bad" behaviors. A major goal of Theraplay treatment is to help caregivers consistently give safety messages to their children and co-regulate their emotions. This is impossible to achieve without empathy for a child's inner life.

By suggesting many possibilities about a child's feelings, needs and intentions, we help caregivers develop compassion for their child in the midst of difficult or confusing behavior. Video review offers many chances to support the caregiver's development of a compassionate "why" behind defensive child behaviors. We gently and repeatedly connect the observed behaviors to the redeeming narrative: the family's history, the child's diagnosis, blocked trust and blocked care, sensory challenges and so on. Helping the caregiver hold an explanation in mind strengthens their ability to maintain empathy for their child—even in the face of very challenging behavior.

In addition to video review, we build reflective functioning through experiential work with caregivers. We deepen self-awareness through practicing Theraplay activities one on one. As the practitioner demonstrates a check-up and places a band-aid on the caregiver's finger, the mother's eyes well with tears. The practitioner reflects her sadness in her own face and body language for a few moments in silence, then says, "Something about this feels a bit sad." The mother nods and seems on the brink of words. "What comes up for you?" We emotionally attune to caregivers, organize their feelings, and support exploration of their inner life.

Scaffolding skills with caregivers for lasting success

At the end of Theraplay treatment, caregivers successfully guide an entire play session with minimal support from us. This is quite an incredible feat. How do we get here? We model, review, scaffold and coach "the Theraplay way" every chance we get.

Initially, the caregiver's role is to follow our lead. We take full responsibility for providing their child with adequate nurture, engagement, structure and challenge and for responding to difficult behavior. This relieves caregivers of shame and anxiety. Protected from the stress of repetitive conflict or attachment rupture, caregivers can focus on their child's perspective, think creatively and respond with new flexibility.

Caregivers benefit greatly from witnessing our therapeutic relationship with their child as it unfolds. As they see us struggle to understand their child, as they observe our failed efforts, uncertainty and frustration, caregivers grow in self-compassion. As our effective strategies take root, caregivers take notice. For months, the caregiver will watch us set firm limits and appropriate developmental challenges, offer co-regulating strategies and not worry about sharing, sportsmanship, fairness or being a "good listener," all to the relationship's benefit. The caregiver will enjoy our calm confidence, our lightheartedness and our sensitive attunement.

Well into treatment, caregivers often report that they are beginning to hear our voice, feel our presence or channel our way in small daily interactions with their child. The caregiver has new priorities, a new playfulness and creativity. The "Theraplay way" is internalized on both explicit and implicit levels.

We coach caregivers towards increasing levels of responsibility in play sessions over time. First, we suggest leading just a few well-known activities. Next, we review tapes, cheer on caregivers and offer subtle adjustments. Ultimately, caregivers are ready to guide an entire session. This milestone represents many months of work on growing self-compassion, reappraising the presenting problem, building reflective functioning and developing new caregiving strategies.

Next, we consider aspects of the Theraplay practitioner's use of self in the treatment process.

The practitioner's use of self in Theraplay practice

In Theraplay practice, we are eliciting and working with the affective, non-verbal and right-brained aspects of our clients' presentation using multisensory and playful methods. We are in the moment with children and families as we work with them. We are actively seeking to engage at a deep interpersonal, attuned and empathetic level.

We don't "do" Theraplay to clients, we are "in" Theraplay with people who have come to us for the alleviation of suffering.

The power of Theraplay lies in this active, intentional use of our whole self—body, mind and emotions—in the service of the children and families with whom we work. This "in the moment" relational focus is highly demanding. If we really attune to the people we work with, then at some level we *feel* their distress too.

Direct social engagement via face, voice and body as discussed in this chapter points to the need for each of us as Theraplay practitioners to be kind to our bodies. In really getting to know our own systems of breathing, muscular activation and facial expression, we can both deepen our attunement to clients and be aware of the impact of the work on ourselves. Yoga or mindfulness practices can give the practitioner a positive way to engage more deeply with these aspects of their professional use of self in Theraplay.

Both traditional attachment theory and modern attachment theory emphasize the importance of the infant being attuned to by their primary caregiver, although Bowlby doesn't use the term attunement (Bowlby, 1999 [1969]; Schore, 2012). In Theraplay, we follow Bowlby in seeing that the ways in which secure attachment is manifested between child and caregiver is a model for us as practitioners.

Primary caregivers who are deeply tuned into their infants know which cry means hunger or loneliness or a wet bottom. Ask them *how* they know that and we doubt that many could put their finger on what exactly distinguishes one cry from another. They might say, "I just know it in my gut." Sadly, our cultures don't always prize this "maternal" form of knowing and, as practitioners, while our "guts" might take the lead in the session in terms of intuitively responding in the moment, professionally and clinically we need to be able to talk about the process.

Drawing together theory from various neurophysiological literature with a specific focus on polyvagal theory, Dana says that "co-regulation is at the heart of positive relationships... When opportunities for connection are missing, we carry our distress in our nervous system" (2018, p.45). In our experience, because of the way in which we stimulate attachment-seeking behaviors in Theraplay practice, we also activate these co-regulatory systems at cognitive, affective, vagal and visceral levels. This gives us a potential route into deeply understanding the inner world of the people with whom we are working and allows us to design Theraplay sessions that use our digestion of that material to offer back a calmer, safer experience of relationship. When this happens, *we* co-regulate the other. Or, if we don't have the professional mechanisms in place to hold, digest and process the experiences, we end up co-regulated (or co-dysregulated) to the distress of our clients and leave ourselves open to vicarious or secondary trauma as well as reducing our effectiveness as practitioners.

In traditional forms of therapeutic practice, the use of counter-transference as a therapeutic tool has a long history, with arguments that explore its "positive" and "negative" value (Gelso & Hayes, 2007). Having a theory to underpin the way in which we use these felt experiences in Theraplay provides us with structure, which, as we know, underpins a sense of safety, regulation and being organized. When we are touched, moved or unsettled by a session, theory can help us work out how to manage the physical and emotional resonance of being undefensively present.

Damasio (2000) uses the term interoception to describe how we get a sense of change in our internal state. Outside our conscious awareness, changes in our blood flow, viscera and chemical balance lead to actions and behaviors. Marks-Tarlow (2014) develops this idea further using the terms clinical intuition and non-verbal insight. Developing the capacity to direct our attention inside ourselves and then back out to the external interaction—as Schön (2011) suggests, to "reflect on action in action"—is a key skill to help us develop as Theraplay practitioners. Theoretical knowledge of these processes can be developed and integrated into practice via clinical and training supervisions or ongoing professional development. These theories provide us with a protective structure in understanding what is happening in sessions.

The videoing of our Theraplay practice opens many possibilities to work at a deeper level for our clients, through using ourselves as instruments of the work. In sessions, there is so much happening at many different levels that it is nearly impossible to be consciously aware of it all in the moment. Being able to take the video of your session to your supervisor means you can take the time to view the video as a whole and also to stop at specific points to reflect on what may be happening.

Your supervisor may guide you in adopting the body posture of others to deepen an exploration of physical and emotional states. You can pay attention to the fluidity of motion, the vocal tone, the facial expressions, the breathing and the distance between all the participants in the session. Such reflection can deepen our understanding of the meaning of relationship and so lead us to the creation of Theraplay sessions and/or activities to support the therapeutic goals of the work.

This deeply reflective and reflexive stance brings to the forefront of our thinking the idea that our responses may be determined by our own cultural and personal positioning, keeping us attuned to a stance of cultural humility. The social GGRRAAACCEEESSS (Burnham, 2011) is a useful acronym to remind us to consider issues around:

- Gender, Geography

- Race, Religion

- Age, Ability, Appearance

- Culture, Class

- Ethnicity, Education, Employment

- Sexuality, Spirituality, Sexual orientation.

You may well come up with other ideas. These social GGRRAAACCEEESSS are not fixed—the idea is a tool to support our sensitivity towards working with diversity.

To make best use of the self of the practitioner, supervision has to feel containing and unthreatening and the practitioner has to have processed enough of their own attachment history to know how to tease out, with the help of the relationship they have with their supervisor, what aspects of their own attachment story are being activated or what they may intuitively, non-verbally and interoceptively be picking up from the people they are working with. We would suggest that this consultative support needs to continue beyond the initial training supervision because of the uniqueness of the co-regulatory (or co-dysregulatory) processes that can occur in Theraplay.

Forms of Theraplay: dyadic, group and Sunshine Circles

The basic concepts of Theraplay's safety and attachment focus, dimensions, process and sequence apply to dyadic parent-child work, Group Theraplay carried out by mental health professionals in settings with or without parents, and in Sunshine Circles delivered by teachers and other leaders in childcare and education settings. This book contains Theraplay applications for various ages, settings, problems and client configurations. We hope that you are inspired by it as we are!

References

Badenoch, B. (2018). "Safety is the Treatment." In N.S. Porges & D. Dana (eds) *Clinical Applications of the Polyvagal Theory: The Emergence of Polyvagal Informed Therapies* (pp.73–88). New York, NY: W.W. Norton & Company.

Baylin, J. (2017). "Social buffering and compassionate stories: The neuroscience of trust building with children in care." *Australian & New Zealand Journal of Family Therapy, 38*(4), 606–612. Available from https://onlinelibrary.wiley.com/doi/full/10.1002/anzf.1272.

Baylin, J. (2018). "Attachment-Focused Treatment and the Brain: A Neuroscience Perspective." In K. Buckwalter & D. Reed (eds) *Attachment Theory in Action: Building Connection Between Children and Parents* (pp.35–50). Lanham, MD: Rowan & Littlefield.

Baylin, J. & Hughes, D. (2016). *The Neurobiology of Attachment-Focused Therapy: Enhancing Connection & Trust in the Treatment of Children and Adolescents.* New York, NY: W.W. Norton & Company.

Bentzen, M. & Hart, S. (2015). *Through Windows of Opportunity.* London, UK: Karnac Books.

Booth, P.B. & Jernberg, A.M. (2010). *Theraplay: Helping Parents and Children Build Better Relationships through Attachment-Based Play.* San Francisco, CA: Jossey-Bass.

Bowlby, J. (1999) [1969]. *Attachment and Loss: Attachment* (second edition). New York, NY: Basic Books.

Bowlby, J. (1988). *A Secure Base: Parent-Child Attachment and Healthy Human Development.* New York, NY: Basic Books.

Burnham, J. (2011). "Developments in Social GGRRAAACCEEESSS: Visible-Invisible and Voiced-Unvoiced." In I.-B. Krause (ed.) *Mutual Perspectives: Culture and Reflexivity in Systemic Psychotherapy.* London, UK: Karnac Books.

Cozolino, L. (2010). *The Neuroscience of Psychotherapy* (second edition). New York, NY: W.W. Norton & Company.

Damasio, A. (2000). *The Feeling of What Happens: Body Emotion and the Making of Consciousness.* London, UK: Vintage Books.

Dana, D. (ed.). (2018). *The Polyvagal Theory in Therapy: Engaging the Rhythm of Regulation.* New York, NY: W.W. Norton & Company.

Dana, D. & Grant, D. (2018). "The Polyvagal Play Lab." In S. Porges & D. Dana (eds) *Clinical Applications of the Polyvagal Theory: The Emergence of Polyvagal Informed Therapies* (pp.185–206). New York, NY: W.W. Norton & Company.

Dissanayake, E. (2001). "Becoming Homo aestheticus: Sources of aesthetic imagination in mother-infant interactions." *SubStance, 94/95,* 85–103.

Fonagy, P., Gergely, G., Jurist, E. & Target, M. (eds). (2002). *Affect Regulation, Mentalization, and the Development of the Self.* New York, NY: Other Press.

Fonagy, P., Steele, H. & Steele, M. (1991). "Maternal representations of attachment during pregnancy predict the organization of infant-mother attachment at one year of age." *Child Development, 62,* 891–905.

Fromm, E. (1956). *The Art of Loving.* New York, NY: Harper and Row.

Geller, S.M. (2018). "Therapeutic Presence and Polyvagal Theory." In S. Porges & D. Dana (eds) *Clinical Applications of the Polyvagal Theory: The Emergence of Polyvagal Informed Therapies* (pp.106–126). New York, NY: W.W. Norton & Company.

Gelso, C.J. & Hayes, J.A. (2007). *Countertransference and the Therapist's Inner Experience: Perils and Possibilities.* Mahwah, NJ: Lawrence Erlbaum Associates.

Kestly, T.A. (2016). "Presence and play: Why mindfulness matters." *International Journal of Play Therapy, 25*(1), 14–23.

Levine, P.A. (2018). "Polyvagal Theory and Trauma." In S. Porges & D. Dana (eds) *Clinical Applications of the Polyvagal Theory: The Emergence of Polyvagal Informed Therapies* (pp.3–26). New York, NY: W.W. Norton & Company.

Lindaman, S. & Mäkelä, J. (2018). "The Polyvagal Foundation of Theraplay Treatment: Combining Social Engagement, Play and Nurture to Create Safety, Regulation and Resilience." In S. Porges & D. Dana (eds) *Clinical Applications of the Polyvagal Theory: The Emergence of Polyvagal Informed Therapies* (pp.227–247). New York, NY: W.W. Norton & Company.

Mäkelä, J. (2003, Fall/Winter). "What makes Theraplay effective: Insights from developmental sciences." *The Theraplay Institute Newsletter*, 5–7.

Marks-Tarlow, T. (2014). *Awakening Clinical Intuition: An Experiential Workbook for Psychotherapists* (Workbook). New York, NY: W.W. Norton & Company.

Meins, E., Fernyhough, C., Wainwright, R., Das Gupta, M., Fradley, E. & Tuckery, M. (2002). "Maternal mind-mindedness and attachment security as predictors of theory of mind understanding." *Child Development, 73*(6), 1715–1726.

Norris, V. & Lender, D. (2020). *Theraplay: The Practitioner's Guide*. London, UK: Jessica Kingsley Publishers.

Ogden, P. (2018). "Polyvagal Theory and Sensorimotor Psychotherapy." In S. Porges & D. Dana (eds) *Clinical Applications of the Polyvagal Theory: The Emergence of Polyvagal Informed Therapies* (pp.34–49). New York, NY: W.W. Norton & Company.

Porges, S.W. (2011). *The Polyvagal Theory: Neurophysiological Foundations of Emotions, Attachment, Communication, and Self-Regulation*. New York, NY: W.W. Norton & Company.

Porges, S.W. (2015). "Play as Neural Exercise: Insights from the Polyvagal Theory." In D. Pearce-McCall (ed.) *The Power of Play for Mind-Brain Health* (pp.3–7). Available from http://mindgains.org.

Porges, S.W. (2017). *The Pocket Guide to the Polyvagal Theory: The Transformative Power of Feeling Safe*. New York, NY: W.W. Norton & Company.

Porges, S.W. (2018). "Polyvagal Theory: A Primer." In S. Porges & D. Dana (eds) *Clinical Applications of the Polyvagal Theory: The Emergence of Polyvagal Informed Therapies* (pp.106–126). New York, NY: W.W. Norton & Company.

Porges, S.W. & Dana, D. (2018). *Clinical Applications of the Polyvagal Theory: The Emergence of Polyvagal Informed Therapies*. New York, NY: W.W. Norton & Company.

Powell, B., Cooper, G., Hoffman, K. & Marvin, B. (2014). *The Circle of Security Intervention: Enhancing Attachment in Early Parent-Child Relationships*. New York, NY: Guilford Press.

Premack, D. & Woodruff, G. (1978). "Does the chimpanzee have a 'theory of mind'?" *Behavioral and Brain Sciences, 4*, 515–526.

Rostad, W.L. & Whitaker, D.J. (2016). "The association between reflective functioning and parent-child relationship quality." *Journal of Child and Family Studies, 25*(7), 2164–2177. Available from https://link.springer.com/article/10.1007/s10826-016-0388-7.

Schön, D.A. (2011). *The Reflective Practitioner: How Professionals Think in Action.* Farnham, Surrey, UK: Ashgate.

Schore, A.N. (2009). "Right Brain Affect Regulation: An Essential Mechanism of Development, Trauma, Dissociation, and Psychotherapy." In D. Fosha, D. Siegel & M. Solomon (eds) *The Healing Power of Emotion: Affective Neuroscience, Development, and Clinical Practice* (pp.112–144). New York, NY: W.W. Norton & Company.

Schore, A.N. (2012). *The Science of the Art of Psychotherapy.* New York: W.W. Norton & Company.

Schore, A.N. & Marks-Tarlow, T. (2018). "How Love Opens Creativity, Play and the Arts Through Early Right-Brain Development." In T. Marks-Tarlow, M. Solomon & D.J. Siegel (eds) *Play and Creativity in Psychotherapy* (pp.64–91). New York, NY: W.W. Norton & Company.

Siegel, D. (1999). *The Developing Mind: How Relationship and the Brain Interact to Shape Who We Are.* New York, NY: Guilford Press.

Siegel, D.J. (2012). *Pocket Guide to Interpersonal Neurobiology.* New York, NY: W.W. Norton & Company.

Trevarthen, C. & Aitken, K.J. (2001). "Infant intersubjectivity: Research, theory and clinical applications." *Journal of Child Psychology and Psychiatry, 42*(1), 3–48.

Tronick, E.Z. & Beeghly, M. (2011). "Infant meaning-making and the development of mental health problems." *American Psychologist, 66*(2), 107–119.

van der Kolk, B. (2018). "Safety and Reciprocity: Polyvagal Theory as a Framework for Understanding and Treating Developmental Trauma." In S. Porges & D. Dana (eds) *Clinical Applications of the Polyvagal Theory: The Emergence of Polyvagal Informed Therapies* (pp.27–33). New York, NY: W.W. Norton & Company.

Wallin, D.J. (2007). *Attachment in Psychotherapy.* New York, NY: Guilford Press.

Winnicott, D.W. (1963). "The development of the capacity for concern." *Bulletin of the Menninger Clinic, 27*(4), 167.

Chapter 2

Ghosts in the Theraplay Room—Exploring, Considering and Understanding the Impact of a Caregiver's Own History on Theraplay Treatment

Karen Doyle Buckwalter

Introduction

Why would some caregivers come to us for help, seem to be fully endorsing what we are observing and suggesting as new ways to interact with their child, but then be unable to carry out the changes we are discussing and modeling for them? Why are some caregivers clearly invested in therapy and helping their child while at the same time unable to shift the behaviors that contribute to the negative family cycle? Why can they not change their steps when we show them the possibility of a new dance with their child? These are questions I often had in my mind over the years when working with caregivers whose children were in Chaddock's Developmental Trauma and Attachment Program® (DTAP®). Obviously, any behavioral pattern or habit can be difficult to change. However, some caregivers seemed to be blocked from making changes by some sort of barrier invisible to both of us.

Other caregivers who come to our offices, although beleaguered and overwhelmed, soak everything up like sponges and fairly quickly are able to incorporate a different way of viewing and parenting their child. We label those who seem unable to implement what we model in Theraplay as difficult, resistant or complex. These "difficult" caregivers may be eager, sincere and motivated or they may be angry and challenging such as those who are mandated to see us by legal systems. Regardless, both groups seem unable to change their behavior in the caregiver-child relationship. Why is this? These questions led me on a quest to understand such caregivers more deeply. This chapter will apply what I found to the Theraplay process.

Key points

1. *A caregiver's own attachment history will impact the ways they engage in Theraplay.* Often when working with caregivers and children I find that this history is not adequately explored and compassionately considered. Attachment is a relational construct, so the "dance" between the caregiver and child is "the client." Thus, understanding the history of the caregiver as well as the child is the foundation for success in many cases.

2. *The Adult Attachment Interview (AAI) is one tool that can be helpful in understanding a caregiver's history.* The interview unearths unconscious memories and patterns of relating that a caregiver may not readily speak about in a typical assessment process. The AAI highlights synaptic shadows from a caregiver's earliest relationships that are impacting their current relationship with their child.

3. *When giving MIM feedback and in Theraplay treatment, the caregiver's own history must be given the same understanding, curiosity and wonder as are given to their children.* The MIM allows the observation of caregiver-child behavior, but the AAI will give clues as to why a caregiver keeps behaving in certain ways even when the therapist suggests other ways of relating.

4. *Rejection of the caregiver by the child can create "blocks" for caregiving that must be explored with the practitioner in order for the caregiver to overcome them.* Such caregivers can appear cold, distant and rejecting and thus may bring up frustration and judgment in the practitioner. In reality, caregivers are being held hostage by the neurochemistry being triggered in their brain which produces fear and rejection rather than joy and connection.

5. *If a caregiver does not hold internal experiences from their own childhood of sensitive caregiving, they will have difficulty giving this to their children in Theraplay.* It is the task of the Theraplay practitioner to model with the caregiver (perhaps for the first time) the types of experiences the practitioner hopes the caregiver will then be able to provide for their child. The experiential nature of Theraplay provides an opportunity to touch and awaken early experiences a caregiver has had with their own caregivers that may enhance or impede progress in Theraplay. Theraplay provides a way for the caregiver to see, feel and explore what they can't tell you in words.

A caregiver's own attachment history will impact the ways they engage in Theraplay

Since Theraplay is an attachment-based model, a caregiver's own attachment history will impact how they engage in Theraplay and how their child will respond to them both in and outside the sessions. There's no question about this as we know from years of attachment research findings the astounding correlation of 75–80 percent between a baby's Ainsworth Strange Situation Protocol (SSP) classification and a caregiver's AAI classification (Van IJzendoorn & Bakersman-Kraneburg, 1997). Mary Main has remarked that the correlation is likely to be even higher. However, due to the fact that both the SSP and the AAI have complicated coding systems, coder error is likely to lower the actual correlation (Main & Hesse, 2009).

Babies don't respond to their caregivers based only on temperament or physiological states such as being hungry or tired. Research has clearly shown that the way a baby responds to caregivers is shaped by what they have learned will be the most effective approach in gaining the caregiver's attention. Babies are biologically programmed to seek safety and protection from their parent or primary caregivers when afraid. Even as early as one year of age, they are exquisitely aware of what behaviors will increase the likelihood that their caregiver will be available to them when needed. Some babies (avoidant) learn that it's better not to be too needy as that drives caregivers away rather than toward them. Or they might learn, when a caregiver is inconsistently available, that it's best to fuss a lot (ambivalent) and this will increase the odds that they will get what they need (Ainsworth *et al.*, 1978). Some babies with disorganized attachment patterns have learned that a caregiver might be frightened of them (as with caregivers who may have unresolved trauma triggered by the baby's needs) or frightening to them, as with abusive caregivers (Hesse & Main, 1999). Whether frightened or frightening, this creates for the baby what Bateson and colleagues (1956) refer to as a "paradoxical injunction," also known as a double bind. The person who is to protect the baby also is afraid of or harms the baby, creating what is known as a disorganized response, yielding behaviors such as walking towards the caregiver backwards after a reunion from separation. Considering all this, in Theraplay we are compelled to understand and work with caregivers as well as children when seeking to address attachment insecurity. In fact, one could argue that a change in the caregiver response to their child is the higher priority as this will then lead to change in the child.

Ann Jernberg's daughter Julie recalled:

> I remember listening to my mother taking extensive histories of the parents' own attachment background in addition to the child's when she did Theraplay intakes over the phone...she would take pages of notes in shorthand on yellow pads of paper...and then she would tailor the Theraplay sessions with this background in mind... I think the parents' own attachment issues as children were key for her therapeutic decision-making... (Personal communication, 2019)

Likewise, Fraiberg, Adelson and Shapiro's (1975) groundbreaking article "Ghosts in the nursery: A psychoanalytic approach to the problems of impaired infant-mother relationships" revealed in a compelling way how "ghosts" from a caregiver's past may invade the caregiver-child relationship from the very start. Fraiberg and her colleagues were working with a mother who, when referred, was described as a "rejecting mother." Indeed, as they watched a video tape of an early home visit, her baby screamed for five minutes while the mother remained distant and self-absorbed and offered no comfort to her baby. They exclaimed to each other in disbelief, "It's as though this mother does not *hear* her baby's cries!" This prompted the diagnostic question "Why doesn't this mother hear her baby's cries?" As Theraplay practitioners, have we not often asked ourselves this same question in one form or another? Why doesn't this caregiver seem able to respond to their child in a helpful and attuned manner? Why can they not read the cues from their child that seem so obvious to us? Fraiberg and her colleagues (1975) came to realize that the mother's own unresolved traumatic past of abandonment and neglect was being re-enacted with her baby. The therapist of the group then focused her work on a relationship where trust could be built with this mother, who, as a child, did not know trust.

The therapist created safety for the mother to speak about feelings from her childhood that had been deeply walled off but which were clearly impacting her ability to be present for her own child. As the therapist began to offer statements such as "That must have been so hard for you as a little girl, and you had no one to turn to. There was no one to hear your cries," the mother's deeply buried grief began to emerge. When this mother's grief came into the room as part of the treatment process, a remarkable thing happened. The mother began gradually to attune to and hear her own baby's cries in ways she was "closed off" from hearing before. As the therapist began to work with this mother, listening—really hearing—and witnessing her story in a way no one had ever heard it before, things began to shift. The therapist was able to gently help the mother see ways that she was repeating what had happened to her with her own baby. The article concludes, and *this* may be the most important sentence of the article, "When this mother's own cries (from her childhood) are heard she will hear her child's cries" (Fraiberg *et al.*, 1975, p.396).

It is not a question of *if* remnants of a caregiver's relational past will impact the relationship they form with their children but rather will the caregiver be aware of this happening and will you as the practitioner have that awareness? For this reason, I am making the case in this chapter that we are missing crucial aspects of how to help a child with Theraplay if we don't simultaneously hold both the child's and the caregiver's stories.

Many of us have had the unfortunate experience in Theraplay of assuming that a caregiver could do what is asked of them only to be both surprised and perhaps saddened when we find that they are not capable of engaging their child in the way that we are trying to guide them. When we don't know the history of caregivers we work with we may assume fluency in a "language" of attachment they have never experienced, or we may ask them to do something in a Theraplay session we quickly discover they are unable to do. Knowing a caregiver's history allows us to more accurately gauge how soon and to what degree we can engage the caregiver in the Theraplay treatment process. It allows us to better understand how well they know the "language" of attachment and what inner representations they may hold (or not hold in the case above) from their own history.

Barriers to exploring a caregiver's attachment history

As stated previously, it is now part of the Theraplay protocol to do some sort of exploration of a caregiver's history. And yet, as I do Theraplay supervision, I find that this exploration and the caregiver-only Theraplay demonstration session often are not happening. Therefore, it seems important to consider the barriers to implementing these aspects of Theraplay treatment.

Caregivers are here for their child rather than themselves and will balk at having caregiver-only sessions.

When practitioners resist this idea of exploring a caregiver's history, the most common reason they give is that caregivers want immediate help for their child and so will not want to have caregiver-only sessions. In Theraplay, we are already having several upfront sessions with the caregiver with the MIM feedback and caregiver demonstration session. What is being suggested here is at least one additional session to better understand the caregiver. Saying there is no time to do this is akin to saying, when taking a trip, "I don't have time to review a map or consider any roadblocks of how to get to where I am going, I just need to get there." One can choose this approach, but generally it makes the journey harder and you may not arrive at your desired destination in the end.

Overcoming this barrier requires educating the caregiver about Theraplay, attachment and the generational transmission of attachment patterns. In all the years of conducting supervision, I have never once had a practitioner tell me, "I really regret spending that extra time with the caregiver to understand their history before starting treatment." Rather, I hear either that they *wish* they had taken time to do this, or they are very glad they *did* do this. When I persist with the idea of the importance of knowing a caregiver's history, most supervisees report that they now can't imagine doing Theraplay without this exploration. When using an attachment-based model that works with the caregiver-child dyad, there's really no way around the fact that each caregiver's history will matter immensely.

It's not appropriate to ask caregivers questions about their background until I have been working with them longer.

A comprehensive assessment should be completed before any therapy begins. As practitioners, we ask about drug use, trauma, sexuality and many other sensitive topics, so why should one hesitate to ask about how a person was raised, considering how that might impact the way they interact with their children? Assessments are used frequently with people who are not in therapy, or who will not have any ongoing relationship with the person administering the assessment. There does not appear to be evidence suggesting that asking about a caregiver's background will have negative repercussions. In fact, as Steele and Steele (2008a) explain in their book *Clinical Applications of the Adult Attachment Interview*, using an assessment such as the AAI early on with caregivers has major benefits:

- It further solidifies with the parent that you will be working from an attachment-based perspective where the history of both parents and children will have impact and importance.

- Taking the time to ask the parent about their history and their current thoughts about it facilitates the therapeutic alliance.

- Such an interview allows for the uncovering of traumatic experiences and losses that may prevent progress with the parent in Theraplay treatment.

- It gives the therapist a deeper understanding of the parent's internal working model and powerful clues regarding the way a parent's history may impact the parent's attention, emotions and behavior towards their child. This helps the therapist discern what the parent is doing related to the current parent-child relationship and what is repetition of a past relationship pattern that is familiar and easily activated by the child.

Another important reason for asking about a caregiver's history early in treatment is that caregivers are more likely to become defensive about such questions when they are asked later in treatment. Often, a practitioner starts to look at these issues due to lack of progress with the caregiver-child dyad. Exploring a caregiver's history at that point is more likely to feel blaming to the caregiver. They may wonder if you are beginning to think maybe *they* are the "problem" rather than their child.

If the caregiver history is explored early on, and caregivers understand you do this with all families, they won't feel singled out for such inquiry and the practitioner will be able to sensitively consider the impact of the caregiver's history right from the start of treatment.

I am working with caregivers who are very defensive, fragile or unstable and exposing them to the questions about their history might make them upset or possibly terminate treatment.

If a caregiver is so unstable that they can't speak about their history then Theraplay may be contraindicated. Theraplay is close, intimate and at times intense and spontaneous. It also involves a great deal of touch and other attachment-promoting and awakening activities. This produces fertile ground for both transference and countertransference to spring up, which is not advisable with an unstable caregiver. We would all agree it's not a good idea to begin Theraplay with a child whose history we are not familiar with or begin not having done any type of assessment. Should we not have the same standard for the other member of the dyad?

I don't have any training working with adults.

Taking the time to explore the caregiver's history and factoring this into treatment is not the same as doing individual therapy with the caregiver. If needs uncovered in this process suggest that the caregiver would benefit from individual therapy, the Theraplay practitioner can and should refer out for this. In such cases, it can be helpful to have a release to speak to the caregiver's therapist should issues come up that might impact the caregiver-child relationship, and to be sure the individual therapist has some understanding of the work you are doing with the caregiver and child.

How to go about exploring the caregiver's history

Finding out about a caregiver's history can be done in a variety of ways. What seems most effective is to have an additional caregiver-only session that occurs before the MIM feedback session. What is learned in this process can then be woven into the MIM feedback. This can deepen the impact of the MIM feedback session significantly. Below are a variety of techniques that can be used.

Parent reflection questions offered in Theraplay training

The level 1 Theraplay training workbook includes the parent reflection questions, some of which are noted or expanded on below. A practitioner could ask a caregiver these questions in a caregiver-only session, or ask caregivers to write out the answers and bring them in for their next appointment. It is recommended that this be done after the initial session with the caregivers so that the practitioner has the information to review when preparing MIM feedback and the caregiver-only Theraplay demonstration session.

Questions about the caregiver's childhood:

- What was it like growing up in your family?

- What types of discipline were used by your caregivers?

- How was your relationship with each of your caregivers similar or different?

- If you were upset as a child, what did you do?

- If you were sick or injured as a child, what did you do?

- Did you lose anyone close to you as a child, either by some sort of separation or death?

- Did you have any experiences as a child you would describe as abusive or traumatic?

- Were there any other adults in your life whom you often turned to for support as a child?

Questions about the present caregiver-child relationship:

- How do you feel when you are with this child?

- Does this child remind you of anyone?

- Do you feel rejected by this child and does that awaken other rejections you have experienced in the past?

- Are there specific behaviors related to your caregiving that you want to change or do more of?

Use of the Adult Attachment Interview (AAI)
to gain understanding of a parent's history

The AAI (George, Kaplan & Main, 1996), which can be obtained online, includes questions about the caregiver's childhood relationship with their caregivers as well as any abusive experiences and significant losses (e.g., the death of people the interviewee was close to and instances surrounding it) in the individual's life. The AAI highlights "synaptic shadows" from a caregiver's earliest relationships that might be impacting their current relationship with their child. To use Fraiberg's metaphor, the AAI allows potential "ghosts in the nursery" to become visible. If the entire interview is used, this may require two additional caregiver sessions rather than only one. The interview often takes more than an hour. Ideally, it would be given in one session that could be extended as long as needed to complete the interview.

Caregiver work beyond initial caregiver-only sessions

The current Theraplay protocol recommends caregiver-only sessions every fourth Theraplay session to review treatment videos and discuss progress related to the initial presenting issues with the child. If this does not happen, caregivers tend to get confused as to why Theraplay is helpful for their child. A caregiver may think "How is blowing bubbles with my child going to help them with being aggressive toward other children?" or "How will feeding my child a snack impact the defiant behavior that brought us to therapy?" Viewing and discussing session videos is very important for helping caregivers gain deeper understanding of the therapy process and for improving their mentalization capacity.

General reflective questions to use while looking at videos

- What seems most interesting to you about this segment?

- What do you like most about what you are doing here?

- Looking at this video now, is there anything you would change in what you are doing?

- What do you like most about what your child is doing?

- What do you like least about what your child is doing?

- Here your child seems to be responding to the structure you are setting. Is that what you are seeing also? Are there other things that appear to be better or worse in the video than when we first started? (Here the practitioner has the option of thinking back to the original presenting problems and MIM feedback to consider what to target in the video review.)

Using caregiver video review to improve mentalization capacity

The concept of mentalization was first developed by Peter Fonagy, Howard Steele, Miriam Steele and others in the 1990s (Fonagy *et al.*, 1991; see also Fonagy, 2008) and has two aspects. The first is the ability to distinguish and find language for one's own subjective states—one's thoughts, feelings, intentions, body sensations—as well as the links between these and how one acts in the world. The other is the ability to generate ideas about the subjective states of another: their thoughts, feelings and so on, and probable links with their behavior in the world. The first aspect we might call "self-mentalization"; the second, "other-mentalization" (Downing, 2016). It is easy to see why mentalization capacity would have a strong impact on caregiving as it allows the caregiver to be aware of their own emotional states and to understand the mind of their child.

An elaborate research instrument, reflective function, or RF, gave meaning and precision to the concept (Fonagy *et al.*, 1991; Steele & Steele, 2008b). RF is a system for coding spoken discourse and was inspired by, and in part derived from, the Adult Attachment Interview (Main, 2008; Main & Goldwyn, 1984). In short, reflective functioning is the operationalization of mentalization. Both self- and other mentalization can be powerful aspects of video review in caregiver-only Theraplay sessions. George Downing (2016), in his work with video intervention therapy, describes a variety of ways video offers unparalleled opportunities for work with mentalization. Describing all of them is beyond the scope of this chapter; however, I will highlight below a few strategies useful in caregiver-only Theraplay sessions when reviewing a video.

Reflective functioning refers to the essential human capacity to understand behavior in light of underlying mental states and intentions

Use of basic mentalization-based questions

A caregiver is sitting with the practitioner looking at a video. On the screen, the caregiver is interacting with their child in a Theraplay session. During this interaction, what might be going on with the caregiver or child? What are the caregiver or child's thoughts, feelings and intentions? How are they reacting to the other? Answers to these mentalization-based questions can readily be explored by the caregiver and the therapist. The video can be stopped at any point, giving a still image of the caregiver and child which provides a compelling point of reference. What at this moment might be going on inside the child? What might have been going on during the preceding seconds? The caregiver and the practitioner can now take time to consider thoughts and ideas about this (Buckwalter & Downing, 2017; Downing, 2008, 2016).

Simple review and reflection—practitioner leading

The practitioner might comment: "As I am watching you and your child playing with bubbles, your child's face seems to show he is delighted. Is that what you are seeing in his face too?"; or, "Are there other times you see this expression from your child?"; or, "If you put yourself back in the moment, what were you thinking and feeling when he had that expression on his face?"

Simple review and reflection—caregiver leading

Therapist: "Hmm, as this bubble playing moves along, his expression and laugh seem to be changing a bit [therapist commenting on external behavior of the child only]. What do you suppose is happening inside him here?"

Giving a voice

Giving a voice (Downing, 2016) is a technique adapted for older children based on the "Speaking for the Baby" program (Carter, Osofsky & Hann, 1991). Here the process is somewhat similar but the caregiver or practitioner is asked to speak as though they were the child. In using the example above:

Therapist: "Hmm, as this bubble playing moves along, his expression and laugh seem to be changing a bit. Imagine you are him. What do you think he might be saying to you right here if he was speaking to you?"

Caregiver: "That high-pitched giggle usually means he's getting overly excited. Maybe he would say, 'Mom, this is really fun but I am starting to feel a bit out of control.'"

Therapist: "Ahh, I see what you are saying there. Yes, that seems likely."

There are endless possibilities for employing this technique when viewing a session video with a caregiver. The discussion could also be extended to discuss what you and the caregiver are learning that helps the child calm down when he starts having his high-pitched giggle, and how this is a cue to watch for from him.

CASE ILLUSTRATION

A mother and father with a pre-teen daughter adopted from China were referred to Chaddock's In-Home Intensive Program. The family was reporting extreme emotional dysregulation from their daughter which sometimes included episodes where she became so angry she would throw things at the parents. The parents also reported extreme defiance and refusal to follow parent directives.

COMMENTS FROM PARENT PAPERWORK ABOUT THEIR OWN HISTORY

From mother: In my home, we were not allowed to show any sort of strong emotion. My mother was an alcoholic. Other than when my mother was drinking, emotions were not expressed much. My father was gone a lot and my mother was preoccupied with her drinking. As a result, I had zero rules and pretty much did as I pleased.

From father: My parents fought a lot and I often recall just trying to stay out of their way. I also was often demeaned and ridiculed by my parents, so I got very good at hiding and controlling my feelings. As I got older, I tried to play the role of peacemaker when there was any sort of family conflict.

In the above parents' MIM, we saw that the parents habitually gave nearly all decision making over to the child. They both appeared conflict avoidant and passive, and both parents lacked the ability to set structure in the MIM. From these observations, we began to wonder if lack of structure and boundaries was contributing to the problems their daughter was presenting.

When giving MIM feedback, we must consider *both* the parent and the child's history. The MIM allows the observation of parent-child behavior, but the information about the parent's background will give clues about why a parent is behaving in specific ways.

In the feedback session with the father, we were able to show him how lost and confused his daughter seemed when he was always asking her what to do next. As the MIM progressed, his daughter appeared increasingly anxious. In pointing this out, we were also able to add empathy and promote insight by stating, "It must be very hard for you to know how to take charge of situations with your daughter after you were conditioned in your family to just be passive, avoid conflict and accommodate. I can imagine you don't even know what taking charge in a situation like this would look or feel like." The father nodded, became tearful and said, "Yes, that's true. I never thought about it that way. I have just felt like I am a bad father and too weak to be what I need to be for my family."

The mother in this family also struggled to provide structure because when she was her daughter's age she simply tried to remain scarce. She had no one to speak with and did her own thing. With no experience with rules or boundaries, the mother did not know what limits to set or how to set them with her daughter, which was clearly evidenced in the MIM and in other information she shared with us. We were able to talk with this mother about the need for limits and boundaries as we watched aspects of the MIM where her daughter took over and began giving her orders. Knowing about the mother's own history allowed us to add empathy and promote awareness about why she struggled so much with setting limits. We discussed how, having grown up in a family where this was not modeled, it would be hard to do in her own family! The mother stated, "I have thought sometimes how my background impacted my marriage, but until this discussion I never considered how my background might be impacting my parenting."

This was a devoted and well-meaning family. They had read many books about parenting children who had experienced early abuse and neglect in orphanage care. They thought they were following what these books said to do, and they were also working with a therapist. However, their history created blind spots and weaknesses in their parenting that they were not able to recognize and therefore were unable to ask for help with. Their lack of ability to set limits and structure with their daughter led to her taking over and doing what she wanted to do. Then, on the rare occasions they did make specific requests they wanted her to comply with, she rebelled and they both retreated. In helping the parents to see this pattern and why, based on their history (and not only the child's behavior), they behaved in this way, we were able to help the parents make changes.

In Theraplay, we have at our disposal such powerful tools with video of the MIM and Theraplay sessions. Both forms of video can be even more potent when we add an understanding of the caregiver's own history and can gently illuminate the places in the relationship where the caregiver is not conscious of how they are contributing to their child's challenges. We have the opportunity to make the unconscious conscious for the caregiver when we have the pieces of the puzzle from their past. Once this is in their conscious, they no longer are held captive to ineffective patterns and we can work with them in Theraplay to change those patterns.

Conclusion

Although Theraplay recommends exploring the caregiver's history, many practitioners do not ask caregivers the reflective questions described above, often citing the caregiver's sense of urgency for the practitioner to start working with their child. Although this allows the practitioner to begin direct work with the child more quickly, the quality of that work is lower than if this additional time with caregivers is taken to explore their history at the start of treatment. What a practitioner learns in doing this will save time in the long run. The narrative the practitioner learns from this process will inform overall treatment in profoundly important ways and it is an essential part of assessment when working from an attachment-based perspective. Don't give in to the pressure from a caregiver or even within yourself to move forward without this information. We must remember that when we work from an attachment-based theoretical orientation, the client is the caregiver-child *relationship*, not only the child. To understand how that relationship functions and remains in stuck and unhelpful patterns, one must understand what both the caregiver and child are bringing to the relationship.

To borrow from trauma expert Bonnie Badenoch's phrasing (Badenoch, 2008), what feelings are touched and awakened (as opposed to triggered) in a caregiver when they are with their child? Many of our earliest memories with caregivers are implicit and not readily reported to a practitioner. Such memories are unconscious, often expressed by the body (tightness on one's chest or an urge to flee from a situation) and show up in ongoing patterns in both our caregiver-child and romantic relationships. Just as we help children to be aware of and label this in Theraplay, with comments such as "Oh, it seems that you are not too sure about this. I can tell by the way you just raised your eyebrows at me," we must do the same for caregivers we work with. Some of this can be done in the actual Theraplay session, but at other times this is best done in our caregiver-only sessions.

John Bowlby (2005) taught that the therapist must become the safe haven and a secure base for a patient to explore their life and consider new ways of being. We need to be this for the caregiver with the hope that they can then be a safe haven and secure base for their child. How can we expect caregivers who have no embodied memories of experiences of attunement and sensitive care from their parents to give this kind of care to their children? The experiential nature of Theraplay provides a unique opportunity to explore and activate experiences a caregiver has had with their own caregivers that may enhance or impede progress in Theraplay. Theraplay provides a way for the caregiver to see, feel and explore what they may be missing from their own attachment history.

Questions for reflection and continued learning

1. How are you assessing the attachment history of caregivers you work with?

2. How are you incorporating the history of both the caregiver and the child you are working with into the MIM analysis, feedback and Theraplay treatment?

3. How are you continuing to work to increase mentalization (both self and other) with caregivers in caregiver-only sessions over the course of Theraplay treatment?

References

Ainsworth, M.D.S., Blehar, M.C., Waters, E. & Wall, S.N. (1978). *Patterns of Attachment: A Psychological Study of the Strange Situation*. Hillsdale, NJ: Erlbaum.

Badenoch, B. (2008). *Being a Brain-Wise Therapist: A Practical Guide to Interpersonal Neurobiology* (Norton Series on Interpersonal Neurobiology). New York, NY: W.W. Norton & Company.

Bateson, G., Jackson, D.D., Haley, J. & Weakland, J. (1956). "Toward a theory of schizophrenia." *Behavioral Science, 1*, 251–254.

Bowlby, J. (2005). *A Secure Base: Clinical Applications of Attachment Theory* (Vol. 393). East Sussex, UK: Brunner-Routledge.

Buckwalter, K. & Downing, G. (2017). "Slowing Down the Dance: Use of Video Intervention Therapy with Parents and Children." In K. Buckwalter & D. Reed (eds) *Attachment Theory in Action* (pp.131–142). Lanham, MD: Rowman and Littlefield.

Carter, S., Osofsky, J. & Hann, D. (1991). "Speaking for the baby: A therapeutic intervention with adolescent mothers and their infants." *Infant Mental Health Journal, 12*, 291–301.

Downing, G. (2008). "A Different Way to Help." In A. Fogel, B. King & S. Shanker (eds) *Human Development in the 21st Century: Visionary Ideas from Systems Scientists* (pp.200–205). Cambridge, UK: Cambridge University Press.

Downing, G. (2016). "Work with Mentalization in Video Intervention Therapy (VIT): Help for Children, Adolescents, and their Parents." In F. Lambruschi & F. Lionetti (eds) *Strumenti di Valutazione e Interventi di Sostegno Alla Genitorialita* (pp.211–232). Rome: Carocci.

Fonagy, P. (2008). "The Mentalization-Focused Approach to Social Development." In F. Busch (ed.) *Mentalization: Theoretical Considerations, Research Findings, and Clinical Implications* (pp.3–56). New York, NY: Analytic Press.

Fonagy, P., Steele, M., Steele, H., Moran, G.S. & Higgitt, A.C. (1991). "The capacity for understanding mental states: The reflective self in parent and child and its significance for security of attachment." *Infant Mental Health Journal, 12*(3), 201–218.

Fraiberg, S., Adelson, E. & Shapiro, V. (1975). "Ghosts in the nursery: A psychoanalytic approach to the problems of impaired infant-mother relationships." *Journal of the American Academy of Child Psychiatry, 14*(3), 387–421.

George, C., Kaplan, N. & Main, M. (1996). "Adult Attachment Interview Protocol" (third edition). Unpublished manuscript, University of California, Berkeley.

Hesse, E. & Main, M. (1999). "Frightened Behavior in Traumatizing but Non-Maltreating Parents: Previously Unexamined Risk Factor for Offspring." In D. Diamond & S.J. Blatt (eds) *Psychoanalytic Theory and Attachment Research I: Theoretical Considerations. Psychoanalytic Inquiry, 19,* 27–38.

Main, M. (2008). "Studying Differences in Language Usage in Recounting Attachment History: An Introduction to the AAI." In H. Steele & M. Steele (eds) *Clinical Applications of the Adult Attachment Interview* (pp.31–68). New York, NY: Guilford Press.

Main, M. & Goldwyn, R. (1984). "Adult Attachment Classification System." Unpublished manuscript, University of California, Berkeley.

Main, M. & Hesse, E. (2009). *Adult Attachment and the Adult Attachment Interview.* Lecture given at Lifespan Learning Institute's Annual IPNB Conference, Los Angeles, CA.

Steele, H. & Steele, M. (eds). (2008a). *Clinical Applications of the Adult Attachment Interview.* New York, NY: Guilford Press.

Steele, H. & Steele, M. (2008b). "On the Origins of Reflective Functioning." In F. Busch (ed.) *Mentalization: Theoretical Considerations, Research Findings, and Clinical Implications* (pp.133–158). New York, NY: Analytic Press.

Van IJzendoorn, M.H. & Bakersman-Kraneburg, M.J. (1997). "Intergenerational Transmission of Attachment: A Move to the Contextual Level." In L. Atkinson & K.J. Zucker (eds) *Attachment and Psychopathology* (pp.135–170). New York, NY: Guilford Press.

Chapter 3

Prenatal and Infant Theraplay

Saara Salo and Hanna Lampi

Introduction

The transition to parenthood is a life-changing process. Future parents go through identity changes, turning more inward into caregiving and nurture and taking care of their close family relationships. The couple's romantic relationship broadens to cover the co-parenting of the joint baby. Self- and other representational changes also include revisiting their own attachment histories, as pregnancy activates memory systems from their own caretaking history. Future parents need to evaluate what good they want to bring into the new relationship with their baby (and what to avoid). This chapter will look at the benefits of Theraplay prenatally and in infancy and toddlerhood.

Key points

1. Emotional attachment to the unborn child starts already during pregnancy and is predictive of later parent-infant attachments. Fetal attachment includes being able to feel positively towards the baby and parenting, the need for protecting and comforting the baby and preparing and making adjustments in one's own life to be ready. Theraplay offers unique ways of helping parents emotionally connect with the unborn child using experiential activities, such as singing and touching, together with reflective talk about how to prepare for parenthood.

2. Anxiety and pre- and postnatal depressive symptoms are very common in the transition to parenthood. They may endanger

the developing relationship with the child. However, empirical evidence has indicated that only treating symptoms of the parents is not enough to ensure that also the parent-child relationship and attachment are improved. Therefore, it has been suggested that interventions should also focus directly on enhancing optimal mother-infant relationships beginning in pregnancy. A randomized controlled study among prenatally depressed mothers using a short-term, manualized prevention model based on Theraplay, called Nurture and Play (NaP), has shown improvements in sensitivity and parental reflectiveness and decreases in depressive symptoms.

3. For the developing social brain, early interaction during the first 12 months is crucial. Infants need sensitively attuned, mirroring and reciprocal connections to be able to develop the necessary skills of joint attention, attachment, emotional regulation and language. Deprivation or misattuned emotional connection can have long-lasting, negative consequences for the child's development. Preliminary research evidence suggests the benefits of Infant Theraplay even in a high-risk sample of mothers with substance-abuse problems.

4. Many babies have difficulties in sleeping, eating and forming daily rhythms during the first year of life. They might have an irritable temperament, including a variety of sensory integration problems. Infant Theraplay offers a practical intervention for helping parents to learn how to be engaged and nurturing, for example how to use touch to calm a fussy baby, or how to structure the daily rhythms of the baby. Helping parents to feel connected to their babies and getting them soothed will eventually lead to more secure attachment by the end of the first year.

5. Babies change family relations between the adult couple and/or in relation to older siblings. Marital dissatisfaction and/or sibling rivalry are typical in the first years of family life with a new baby. Infant Theraplay is often offered as Family Theraplay, including working with the adult couple and/or siblings. Thus, all emotional connections within a family system can be acknowledged.

Theraplay in the prenatal phase
Enhancing early emotional attachment
with Prenatal Theraplay

Adjusting to pregnancy as a physiological state, with bodily and hormonal changes including cognitive changes in attention and memory functions, both facilitates the psychological process of pregnancy but also can cause, at least, occasional stress. All in all, pregnancy is an enormously emotional period for the new parents, with ups and downs in mood, and related cognitive and biological changes. The process of pregnancy helps in developing a new, emotional relationship with the unborn child and preparing for caretaking of the newcomer.

These protective bonding feelings usually emerge after the tenth gestational week. Normally, emotional processing changes during pregnancy, with pregnant women being emotionally more perceptive and open to processing emotional interpersonal signals, especially negative emotions. This may be especially adaptive, given that the newborn baby has very limited capacities of expressing his/her needs besides the distress signals. Furthermore, more recently, the reflective side of prenatal parenting, that is, thinking and imagining the future baby and the relationship, has also been underlined as an important predictor of the future attachment relationship with the actual baby. The prenatal reflectiveness includes the realization that the fetal baby is already a unique, separate human being with feelings separate from the parents (Slade *et al.*, 2009). This reflective capacity paves the way for accurate perception of the child's emotional cues, sensitive responding and the formation of secure attachment of the child during infancy (Camoirano, 2017; Slade *et al.*, 2005).

Unfortunately, pregnancy often is also a very stressful time. Prenatal depression and anxiety problems are increasingly common, with prevalence estimates ranging from 10 to 30 percent (Field, 2011, 2017). These, in turn, have negative effects on the developing emotional attachment with the unborn child. Enhancing the developing emotional relationship with the unborn child seems, therefore, an important intervention goal. However, most early interventions have still focused predominantly on reducing mothers' pre- and postnatal depressive/anxiety symptoms (Lefkovics, Baji & Rigó, 2014), although reducing mothers' depressive symptoms alone does not appear to lead to improvements in parenting or in infant well-being and development (Forman *et al.*, 2007).

Prenatal Theraplay offers a unique possibility of creating new moments of emotionally connecting with the unborn child and reflecting on the process of becoming a parent. In practice, before beginning, we interview the parent(s) about the experience of being pregnant, and do the prenatal MIM, which consists of tasks such as "Sing to your baby," as well as tasks exploring more the reflective parts of the developing relationship, such as "Tell your child about the people he/she will meet." Jernberg, Thomas and Wickersham (1985) described the potential benefits for parents doing the prenatal MIM: "Taking the MIM allows parents the experience of relating to, communicating with, and articulating their hopes and fears about their unborn baby" (p.24). The prenatal MIM also can be used as an intervention tool to follow the process of pregnancy. Thus, redoing some of the MIM tasks later on in the Prenatal Theraplay sessions may give a unique opportunity for the practitioner and the parent to observe changes in representations and related affects and thoughts. In particular, redoing the task "Draw a picture of you and your baby" is likely to reveal changes.

In the Prenatal Theraplay sessions, through playful Theraplay activities, such as singing, touching the tummy baby, measuring and making a foil print of the tummy, and bodily relaxation exercises with the parent (see Salo & Lampi, 2019), the emotional parts of the caregiving system of the parental brain can be stimulated. All these activities are designed especially to promote the engagement and nurture dimensions, through physical touch and reciprocity. The other main dimensions of Theraplay—structure and challenge—are less evident as we are still very much working on an imaginary level. Nevertheless, they are acknowledged in the way the Prenatal Theraplay sessions are carried out using a pre-planned, practitioner-led structure, comprising attachment-based activities and reflective discussions about the feelings and thoughts of the parent. If the parent is experiencing mood-related problems as described above, they have often been shown to have specific problems in sensitive attunement, using less physical touch and in a less affectionate manner, and using more negative vocal behavior and less infant-directed speech (Field, 2010, 2011).

In Prenatal Theraplay, thus, we focus on these affective ways of relating by actively guiding the mothers to participate in the activities in sensitive and responsive ways. Prenatal Theraplay is also a direct way of working reflectively with the unborn child, as the baby is very much a subject in the Theraplay sessions. For example, we direct our speech and singing directly to the unborn child. Finally, prenatal sessions also include reflective discussions with parents about how they currently feel about their pregnancies. As much as possible, the reflective focus is in the present moment, for example what the parent was able to perceive right there and then when singing to the unborn child. The goal is to improve the prenatal reflectiveness, that is, being aware of the baby's responses as separate from one's own.

RCT study on Nurture and Play—a Theraplay-based group for pregnant depressive women

The Prenatal Theraplay-based intervention, called Nurture and Play (NaP), was recently evaluated in a randomized controlled study design by Salo and colleagues (Salo *et al.*, 2019). NaP is a derivative of Theraplay and it utilizes Theraplay-based activities (Poutiainen & Salo, 2015; Salo & Lampi, 2019). NaP was designed to be a short-term, manualized intervention, with training easy to provide in multi-professional settings, and with the main goal of serving as a preventive tool for mothers with prenatal depressive symptoms. As such, besides using Theraplay activities, NaP also covers the mentalized relationship with the baby with the use of special reflective techniques as well as cognitive strategies to deal with the mood-related problems.

Thus, the structure of each NaP session in the study was to strengthen both the emotional and experiential (how the baby is felt, what can be perceived through bodily emotional and somatosensory cues) as well as the imaginary (mentalized) relationship with the baby. NaP was also conducted in a group setting to facilitate the support mothers could get from each other in a similar life situation. The randomized control trial study examined participants (45 women from a community setting, who screened positive for depressive symptoms during pregnancy) who were randomly assigned to the intervention group (n = 24) and a treatment-as-usual group (n = 21). Women in the intervention group participated in the NaP intervention from pregnancy until the baby was seven months of age. The results revealed that the intervention group showed a greater increase in maternal sensitivity and reflective functioning and a greater decrease in depressive symptoms as compared to the control group. These findings provide preliminary support for the effectiveness of the NaP intervention in enhancing early maternal caregiving qualities of maternal reflective functioning and sensitivity as well as decreasing depressive symptoms. The findings also lend support for the Prenatal Theraplay work in general.

Special considerations/adaptations of Theraplay when working in the prenatal phase

Doing Prenatal Theraplay requires an adequate clinical framework where the practitioner is assigned to work with the individual parent's well-being and psychological process of being pregnant. There needs to be enough time to process issues arising during pregnancy, such as health-related issues of the baby, more severe depressive or anxiety symptoms, fear of birth and so on. Knowledge and experience about the psychological and physiological process of pregnancy is needed, as the Theraplay sessions also include much more talk on these subjects than other forms of Theraplay. Furthermore, as Jernberg *et al.* (1985) already describe in their innovative approach to the prenatal MIM, including fathers may be especially relevant. However, here, couple relational issues need to be considered. With highly quarrelsome couples, for example, and the expectant mother experiencing many psychiatric symptoms, including the father in Theraplay sessions might not be possible.

 CASE ILLUSTRATION

Anna, a married 37-year-old secretary expecting her first child, began treatment at gestational week 29. She had told her midwife about not being able to sleep, with anxious thoughts about the baby's well-being and the upcoming birth. She said she was sure that she would miscarry, and she was very worried about the baby's health. She had suffered one miscarriage before at a rather early stage of pregnancy. Anna's midwife consulted the team's psychiatrist, who referred Anna for a visit with a parent-infant psychotherapist/Theraplay practitioner for a prenatal MIM and related MIM interview to make a further treatment plan.

SUMMARY OF TWO TASKS OBSERVED

In the first prenatal MIM task, when asked to draw a picture of her and her baby, Anna drew a smiling mother holding a small baby. She verbally explained to the assessor that the "child is smiling because he sees the mommy's smiling face." She had a warm expression on her face, but also tears in her eyes when talking about the drawing. In another prenatal MIM task where the parent is asked to tell the child first something without words and then with words, Anna placed both her hands firmly on the belly but then pulled them abruptly away, and said that she was trying to check where the baby's head was, but then she suddenly was worried if she couldn't feel the movements, so she stopped.

QUALITATIVE ANALYSIS
The mother's engagement was rather high but ambivalent throughout the MIM; she attuned to the unborn child both affectively by touch and gestures but she was also tearful and pulled away. She was well structured in her manner of proceeding, performing the activities in developmentally feasible ways (challenge), being able to mentalize the child's perspective by checking where the child's head was.

PRENATAL THERAPLAY
In weekly sessions with the Theraplay practitioner, Anna was gently encouraged to try to stay affectively connected with the unborn child as well as encouraged to talk and reflect about her ambivalent feelings. Thus, in the sessions, there was singing, measuring the tummy, using a musical instrument and waiting to see if the unborn child heard and responded, drawing the baby and the mother, and so on. Also, the practitioner led a discussion where Anna's previous miscarriage and understandable fears of becoming attached were explored together. After three sessions, Anna was visibly able to relax more, she oriented towards her unborn child more by using touch and said she experienced fewer sudden worried feelings. The prenatal work continued until gestational week 36. In the last sessions, increasing time was spent on the approaching birth experience; for example, Anna wrote a letter to her newborn baby and prepared her child for birth.

HOME VISIT AFTER BIRTH
The Theraplay practitioner visited the home after the birth, meeting with the mother, father and baby. During this visit, the birth experience and initial settling into living with the baby were discussed with the aim of providing support for the developing emotional relationship with the baby.

INFANT THERAPLAY

Infant Theraplay with baby Stefan and Anna started when Stefan was ten weeks old. In the sessions, the main goal was to further strengthen the engagement. Through singing, baby massaging, making foot prints and measuring Stefan, Anna seemed to enjoy her baby and she was able to read and respond to Stefan's cues. As Anna herself still felt a bit unsure and anxious when Stefan cried, there was a special emphasis on nurture in the sessions. Thus, different holding positions were tried out together, and gentle massaging of the feet and belly, as practical ways Anna could use in their everyday life to help to calm Stefan down. Infant Theraplay continued until Stefan was five months old. By that time, Stefan was developing well and Anna was able to interact with her son in positive and lively ways. The practitioner and mother felt that no further treatment was needed but the mother could access the practitioner with questions or concerns.

Table 3.1: Example activities for Prenatal Theraplay (Salo & Lampi, 2019)

Prenatal Theraplay	Nurture	Engagement	Structure, Challenge
Examples of Theraplay activities	Nurturing mother's hands Relaxation Weather report Back massage	Singing Putting a tape with a "working name" of the baby on mother's belly Playing a musical instrument Measuring the belly Decorating the belly (taking picture)	Exploring the baby's senses with touch, light and music, e.g., playing a musical instrument to the baby and following baby's responses

The developing social brain:
Theraplay in infancy and toddlerhood

Early parent-child interaction—comprising the Theraplay dimensions of structure, engagement, nurture and challenge—has long been associated with a child's later cognitive and socio-emotional development and general well-being. Its role is greatest during infancy, due to the experience-dependent nature of brain development (Greenough, Black & Wallace, 1987), where the developing brain mechanisms are dependent on the social input they get (Atzil, Hendler & Feldman, 2013). For many reasons, parents may have difficulties in early interaction with their babies. Postnatal depression, traumatizing birth experiences and increases in marital dissatisfaction are among the underlying causes that may lead into a withdrawn, non-synchronized pattern of not being able to notice and respond sensitively to the infant's signals (e.g., Field, 2010; Korja *et al.*, 2016; Muller-Nix *et al.*, 2004). Low self-esteem and perceived competence, lack of social support and the parent's own attachment insecurities may also lead to low responding or too intrusive attempts when trying to soothe or engage the baby (e.g., Jones & Prinze, 2005; Mills-Koonce *et al.*, 2011). Furthermore, infants are born with different temperament profiles, with some easier to soothe than others. Infants may also have developmental, regulatory problems that make their feeding and sleeping, and the related parent-child interaction, very difficult (Kim & Kochanska, 2012). The constant caretaking and nurturing of infants can be an enormously stressful period for many parents, with long-lasting influences in the child's development.

Infant Theraplay offers a unique possibility of helping parents directly to notice their infant's signals, and, most importantly, to learn how to synchronize, mirror and regulate their structuring, engaging, nurturing and challenging responses so that these will lead into precious moments-of-meeting with the infant. Again, before the Theraplay sessions, we make an individually tailored treatment plan for each parent-child dyad using the MIM and an interview, probing for the relational history and parental representations and reflections about the infant and the current relationship. If we began work with the family prenatally, we may not administer the MIM postnatally. The parent and infant are together with the practitioner in weekly sessions for approximately 15–20 times, either at the clinic or in their home.

Infant Theraplay sessions include a similar structure as working with older children. We start by welcoming and checking activities, for example checking the eye color of the infant/parent dyad, measuring the infant, making foot prints and so on. Playful activities such as watching/catching soap bubbles, using various rhythmic movements and singing are used in the middle parts of the session, and we end with more soothing activities such as rocking the baby and singing a lullaby. As infants have their own feeding rhythm, we don't necessarily end with feeding, especially with breast-feeding infants. Certainly, if the infant is hungry at any point of the session, we need to take a pause for feeding. With older babies and toddlers, adding a healthy snack is usually part of the ending activities, as with older children. During the sessions, the practitioner actively wonders aloud what the infant might be feeling and experiencing and tries to involve the parent in this wondering. Adult emotional and behavioral responses and modifications to the Theraplay activities are actively linked to these wonderings, for example by empathetically responding that some activities might have been too strong for the infant ("Let's do it again more softly") and helping the parent to adjust their response.

There is much focus on achieving a level of embodied relations (e.g., using "Row-row-row a boat" mirroring the muscular strength or affective expression on the infant's face). We also use a surprise-activating element behind all the activities designed to promote joint attention and to arouse positive feelings (e.g., peek-a-boo). As attachment theory highlights, the parent's ability to detect and accurately respond to the infant's signs of stress is important in the development of internalized stress-regulatory capacity. The biochemical mechanisms explaining this link have been shown to involve oxytocin, which in turn is related to the provision of maternal touch underlying the basic bonding mechanism (Apter-Levy *et al.*, 2013). We help the parents, for instance finding ways of calming an over-active or restless child by helping the child accept soothing physical closeness and touch. As well as increasing the amount of touch, the maternal (or paternal) affectionate style of using touch has been found to be of importance. Thus, we increase maternal touch not by verbal instructions but rather by doing activities together, with the practitioner and the parent side by side. Finally, we support the parents' ability to offer positive guidance by coaching them to directly guide, encourage and help the infant in problematic situations. This occurs in games that are designed to reinforce the infant's self-confidence through success, such as letting a five-month-old grasp soap bubbles from the air themselves.

As parents are active participants in Infant Theraplay sessions, there is a special need for planning separate video reflections. Thus, after starting

Theraplay, there are separate video reflections with the parents after every third session where parental reflectiveness is supported by helping the parents see and feel situations from the child's and their own perspective. There are three goals in this work:

- Increasing parental attention to the child's emotional and behavioral signals during interaction.

- Focusing on parental feelings and thoughts about the interaction: "Will I be able to have a satisfying and sustainable emotional engagement with the baby?"

- Recognizing those interactional patterns and infant responses that are healthy and show developmental progress.

Special considerations/adaptations of Infant Theraplay working with families

With infants, a special emphasis is keeping the dyadic focus—that is, holding the infant and parent in our minds together. Thus, we keep the parent/infant dyad together as much as possible, the parent holding the infant and performing as many of the activities as they can. We constantly make links between them, so the focus is less intensely on the events between infant and the practitioner (e.g., commenting "I see you have blue eyes, just like your mom"). The purpose is to immediately reinforce the developing parental competence and to avoid the parental feelings that the practitioner is better at engaging the infant. We also need enough understanding of infant development to plan and execute the sessions so that they will promote the infant's current development, for instance knowing when infants can reach for objects, sit up on their own or mirror/copy movements. Practitioner experience in working with infants and updated knowledge on various developmental issues, including feeding and sleeping, is also needed. If there are any special needs or worries about the infant's development (lack/avoidance of eye contact, clear problems in cognitive or motor functioning), these need to be addressed, not only in adjusting Theraplay activities but also when generalizing the result into everyday life.

Family Theraplay addresses emotional connections within the family system

Finally, using Family Theraplay might be especially warranted during infancy. In many couples, marital satisfaction declines due to daily hassles, sleep deprivation and the stressful struggles new parents face when trying to combine work-related pressures and so on with the needs of a young child. Furthermore, if there are older siblings in the family, they will inevitably react to the birth of a younger sibling. Normative sibling rivalry and feelings of being excluded are expected changes in the family dynamics. In many cases, parents struggle to adjust to these changes, and their interaction quality with each other and/or older siblings may suffer. Doing Family Theraplay sessions, where everyone takes part and the children all receive parental attention, has proven to be helpful here. In Family Theraplay, the practitioner leads the sessions, helping the parents to guide their children. All children receive nurture and engagement, and structuring and challenging activities can be modified so all family members can take part, even when they are developmentally in different phases. For example, adding three to four Family Theraplay sessions at the end of the Infant Theraplay process has been shown to increase the emotional cohesion and bonding between all family members, not just the infant and parent. For example, in a family measuring activity, the practitioner measures a foot or finger of the older sibling and then helps the child to measure the mom, dad and baby; measurements can be recoded for comparison as the children grow.

 ## CASE ILLUSTRATION: TODDLER

Stella was 12 months of age when she and her parents, Peter and Maria, started Theraplay. Stella had been a fussy baby, having difficulties in sleeping and feeding from early on. Still she slept very lightly, startling easily, and she needed carrying and comforting to be able to get back to sleep. She had had a hard time getting used to solids and was a fussy eater, which worried her parents. They also described Stella as a timid child, and there were only a few close family members with whom Stella was comfortable, and only for a short period of time. She was easily overwhelmed in new situations and even positive events often ended in a temper tantrum. Her parents recounted that she was easily startled by loud noises and did not like roughhousing or other more active forms of playing. Stella was about to start daycare and the parents were worried about how she would adjust and wished for support and help.

In the family MIM, the parents were very sensitive and caring towards Stella. They had difficulties directing her or asking her to do something she didn't want to. In these situations, Dad was quicker to try to adjust the situation according to what he thought were Stella's wishes, as Mom was still trying to continue in a more adult-led way. After the MIM and feedback session, the parents had their own Theraplay demo session and 15 Theraplay sessions, including the video feedback work with parents. The goals for Theraplay were to help Stella engage with more people, to help the parents challenge Stella and to find ways to help Stella regulate in difficult situations. The parents also wished to have time to discuss their co-parenting in the process.

Both parents and Stella were present at all Theraplay sessions. In the beginning, Stella was quieter and more subdued in the sessions. She enjoyed nurturing activities and joined in new activities after she was shown them with Mom or Dad first. Little by little, her confidence grew, and after five sessions she was readier to accept new activities without first seeing them done by her parents. We focused on building the challenge and structure and chose the activities accordingly. In parent feedback sessions, we discussed how parents had different views on how many demands Stella could take. Mom was frustrated at times since she felt that Dad undermined her efforts to encourage Stella to taste new foods and try new things. Both parents saw that in Theraplay sessions Stella was able to overcome initial shyness as the adult was staying positive and persistent with her. With her parents, strategies were planned to make meal times more fun and they thought about ways to boost her self-confidence. By the end of the Theraplay process, Stella had started at daycare, and even though she was still slow to warm up to new people, she had started to build trusting relationships with the staff. The parents felt that they had acquired confidence in their parenting in the process, and as Stella had grown they found it easier to meet her age appropriately.

Table 3.2: Example activities for Toddler Theraplay (Salo & Lampi, 2019)

Toddler Theraplay	Nurture	Engagement	Structure, Challenge
Examples of Theraplay activities	Songs (welcome song, ending song) Lotion Blanket swing Feeding	Bean-bag drop Measuring Blowing a cotton ball Stack of hands	Soap bubbles Push me down, pull me up Stop and go Crawling race

Pre- and post-study on Infant Theraplay among mothers with substance abuse disorder (SUD)

Parental substance abuse has serious implications for the later development of the child, with an increased risk for emotional and physical neglect, and academic, social and emotional problems of the infant (Salo & Flykt, 2013). In Finland, there are 13 special units designed for pregnant and parenting women who have severe substance abuse problems. These units are part of the child protection field in the social and welfare sector (Federation of Mother and Child Homes and Shelters; the treatment program is called "Hold On") (Pajulo *et al.*, 2006). The intensive treatment lasts about one year and comprises both psychosocial as well as necessary medical interventions (detoxication and other medical or mental health treatment if needed). As many substance-abusing mothers lack the basic capability of affect reading, interpretation and responding to their children's emotional signals, often related to their own disturbed and traumatic attachment histories (Lyden & Suchman, 2013), we conducted a pilot study in this setting to evaluate the feasibility and impact of Infant Theraplay (Salo, 2011).

Seven mother-infant pairs participated in Infant Theraplay and six mother-child pairs served as matched controls receiving everything else in the treatment except Theraplay. The mean age of the mothers was 29.7 (standard deviation 4) and the infants 12.3 months (standard deviation 7.7). MIM assessment and interviews assessing maternal representations or reflective functioning were conducted before and after Theraplay. Most mothers had used intravenous drugs for several years. Thirty-nine percent of the mothers had experienced their own parents' substance abuse during childhood and 23 percent had been in foster placement. Their interaction in the first MIM showed that there were significant problems in sensitivity (e.g., showing positive emotions) and intrusiveness (e.g., reading the child's initiatives and readiness for interaction). These facts were taken into consideration when planning the Infant Theraplay sessions by using a specific "trauma lens" as suggested by Lieberman and Amaya-Jackson (2005).

Thus, due to distortions in the mother's own attachment system and related reflective capabilities, there may be a lack of maternal procedural capabilities in using her hands, heartbeat, rhythm, singing, rocking and so on as soothing interpersonal devices for the child even when the parent is able to detect the child's emotional signs of distress. Adopting a "trauma lens" may help the therapist to take special care in being predictable and clear and avoiding too much intensity, especially when working with an active form of therapy such as Theraplay. The results showed that there was a statistically significant improvement in maternal sensitivity—for example, the mother's ability to express positive emotions and respond accurately to the infant's behavioral cues—and creativity in play in those mothers participating in Theraplay as compared with mothers who did not receive Theraplay (Salo, 2011). It may be that Theraplay activities that really felt fun and engaging to the parent made the interaction altogether more enjoyable with the infant. The positive feedback given in the video reflections and the overall warm, supportive attitude of the Theraplay practitioner towards the mother may have helped the mother to both experience and express more positive feelings towards the child. The overall positive experiences of utilizing Infant Theraplay as a part of the rehabilitation, especially in increasing maternal sensitivity, have led to its systematic and ongoing use in both residential settings and open care units over the past ten years.

Conclusion

Prenatal and Infant-Toddler Theraplay serve to strengthen the emotional bond between a parent and the child, even starting before birth. From a preventive perspective this is especially important, as many parents suffer from an increase in psychiatric symptoms, including depressive and anxiety problems, marital dissatisfaction and lack of social support, which put the child's attachment development at risk. Furthermore, among different early interventions, Theraplay is unique in its capability of directly focusing on the emotional experience of becoming a parent. Focusing directly on attunement, mirroring, synchrony and mutuality as well as developmentally appropriate structure and guidance, Theraplay is in line with current theories and understanding of what constitutes the basis for optimal socio-emotional development. Furthermore, in Theraplay, the parental side of being able to reflectively understand the new role of being a mother/father as well as the dynamics of the relationship is demonstrated in the program in the active use of video reflective work. Helping parents to feel more competent and secure in emotionally attuning and responding to their child's needs as well as developing their related reflective skills to support these behavioral capabilities will have long-lasting consequences for the child. There is preliminary empirical support for Prenatal and Infant Theraplay, or its variant the NaP intervention, and future studies are being conducted. Finally, taking a family perspective may help in supporting the new role for older siblings.

Questions for reflection and continued learning

1. Why work with the parent-child relationship starting prenatally?

2. What are the two main goals in Prenatal Theraplay?

3. Why is Infant Theraplay important for the baby?

References

Apter-Levy, Y., Feldman, M., Vakart, A., Ebstein, R.P. & Feldman, R. (2013). "The impact of maternal depression across the first 6 years of life on the child's mental health, social engagement and empathy: The moderating role of oxytocin." *American Journal of Psychiatry, 170,* 1161–1168.

Atzil, S., Hendler, T. & Feldman, R. (2013). "The brain basis of social synchrony." *Social Cognitive and Affective Neuroscience, 20,* 2–10.

Camoirano, A. (2017). "Mentalizing makes parenting work: A review about parental reflective functioning and clinical interventions to improve it." *Frontiers in Psychology, 8.*

Field, T. (2010). "Postpartum depression effects on early interactions, parenting, and safety practices: A review." *Infant Behavior and Development, 33,* 1–6.

Field, T. (2011). "Prenatal depression effects on early development: A review." *Infant Behavior and Development, 34,* 1–14.

Field, T. (2017). "Prenatal depression risk factors, developmental effects and interventions: A review." *Journal of Pregnancy and Child Health, 4*(1), 301.

Forman, D.R., O'Hara, M.W., Stuart, S., Gorman, L.L., Larsen, K.E. & Coy, K.C. (2007). "Effective treatment for postpartum depression is not sufficient to improve the developing mother-child relationship." *Development and Psychopathology, 19*(2), 585–602.

Greenough, W.T., Black, J.E. & Wallace, C.S. (1987). "Experience and brain development." *Child Development, 58*, 539–559.

Jernberg, A.M., Thomas, E. & Wickersham, M. (1985). *Mothers' Behaviors and Attitudes Toward their Unborn Infants.* Chicago, IL: The Theraplay Institute.

Jones, T.L. & Prinz, R.J. (2005). "Potential roles of parental self-efficacy in parent and child adjustment: A review." *Clinical Psychology Review, 25*(3), 341–363.

Kim, S. & Kochanska, G. (2012). "Child temperament moderates effects of parent-child mutuality on self-regulation: A relationship-based path for emotionally negative infants." *Child Development, 83*(4), 1275–1289.

Korja, R., Piha, J., Otava, R., Lavanchy-Scaiola, C. *et al.* (2016). "Mother's marital satisfaction associated with the quality of mother-father-child triadic interaction." *Scandinavian Journal of Psychology, 57*(4), 305–312.

Lefkovics, E., Baji, I. & Rigó, J. (2014). "Impact of maternal depression on pregnancies and on early attachment." *Infant Mental Health Journal, 35*(4), 354–365.

Lieberman, A. & Amaya-Jackson, L. (2005). "Reciprocal Influences of Attachment and Trauma: Using a Dual Lens in the Assessment and Treatment of Infants, Toddlers, and Preschoolers." In L. Berlin, Y. Ziv, L. Amaya-Jackson & M.T. Greenberg (eds) *Enhancing Early Attachments* (pp.100–127). New York, NY: Guilford Press.

Lyden, H.M. & Suchman, N. (2013). "Transmission of Parenting Models at the Level of Representation: Implications for Mother-Child Dyads Affected by Maternal Substance Abuse." In N. Suchman, M. Pajulo & L. Mayes (eds) *Parenting and Substance.* New York, NY: Oxford University Press.

Mills-Koonce, W.R., Appleyard, K., Barnett, M., Deng, M., Putallaz, M. & Cox, M. (2011). "Adult attachment style and stress as risk factors for early maternal sensitivity and negativity." *Infant Mental Health Journal, 32*(3), 277–285.

Muller-Nix, C., Forcada-Guex, M., Pierrehumbert, B., Jaunin, L., Borghini, A. & Ansermet, F. (2004). "Prematurity, maternal stress and mother-child interactions." *Early Human Development, 79*(2), 145–158.

Pajulo, M., Suchman, N., Kalland, M. & Mayes, L. (2006). "Enhancing the effectiveness of residential treatment for substance abusing pregnant and parenting women: Focus on maternal reflective functioning and mother-child relationship." *Infant Mental Health Journal: Official, 27*(5), 448.

Poutiainen, T. & Salo, S. (2015). *Nurture and Play: A Group Intervention for Pregnant Mothers. Finnish Handbook.* Lahti: Lahden Diakoniasäätiö.

Salo, S. (2011). "Does Theraplay increase emotional availability among substance-abusing mother-infant dyads?" Oral presentation, ESCAP. *European Child and Adolescent Psychiatry*, Helsinki, 11–15.

Salo, S. & Flykt, M. (2013). "The Impact of Parental Addiction on Child Development." In N. Suchman, M. Pajulo & L. Mayes (eds) *Parenting and Substance Abuse: Developmental Approaches to Intervention* (pp.196–200). New York, NY: Oxford University Press.

Salo, S. & Lampi, H. (2019). *Nurture and Play—Activities for Professionals*. Espoo: TerapiaLampi Inc.

Salo, S., Flykt, M., Mäkelä, J., Biringen, Z. *et al.* (2019). "The effectiveness of nurture and play: A mentalisation-based parenting group intervention for prenatally depressed mothers." *Primary Health Care Research & Development, 20*, E157. doi:10.1017/S1463423619000914.

Slade, A., Cohen, L.J., Sadler, L.S. & Miller, M. (2009). "The psychology and psychopathology of pregnancy." *Handbook of Infant Mental Health, 3*, 22–39.

Slade, A., Grienenberger, J., Bernbach, E., Levy, D. & Locker, A. (2005). "Maternal reflective functioning, attachment, and the transmission gap: A preliminary study." *Attachment and Human Development, 7*, 283–298.

Chapter 4

Theraplay with Adolescents

Fiona Peacock

Introduction

Theraplay, modeled as it is on patterns of attachment behaviors between infants and their primary caregivers, might not seem a ready fit for adolescents with those same primary caregivers. No longer can you pick your child up and place them on your lap. Now you stand toe-to-toe with a young person whose feet are bigger than yours and who is so tall that you have to tilt your head up to see them. What a shift! Now we have to literally look up to our babies! How can Theraplay be adapted for working with adolescents?

Key points

1. Without an understanding of typical or atypical development in adolescence, one might mistake normal developmental processes for dysfunctional development.

2. Stimulating attachment behaviors and experiences will help adolescents address the normal challenges of this developmental phase.

3. The core Theraplay model needs to be used flexibly and blended, at times, with other therapeutic approaches to ensure the needs of the adolescent are met.

4. We need to think carefully about using a relational model of therapeutic intervention for adolescents who have experienced developmental or relational trauma, and make appropriate adaptions.

Developmental tasks of adolescents

We practice Theraplay in many cultural settings, so we need to be mindful of the attitudes and values that we, as well as our clients, might implicitly bring to our work. In the authors' background section I introduced myself from my professional identity. Focusing on adolescents and their specific needs in this chapter, I feel the need to offer a more personal introduction. I write about adolescence as a cisgendered, white, middle-aged English woman who has had the privilege of post-compulsory education, is financially independent and has been raised in a Christo-centric culture that affirms my spiritual roots (Krause, 2002). I write from a place of power, as an educated white adult, but am more comfortable with the idea of "power with" rather than "power over." I write with an interest and aptitude for verbal language knowing I am not a "digital native" and speak that poorly as a second or third language. So, what has all that got to do with making sense of the term "adolescence" and the experience of being adolescent? Is adolescence just a culturally created construct or a universal maturation process?

Examining our own biases around our valuing of this life stage may mean we approach Theraplay with adolescents having an inkling of where the challenges might lie. I find it helpful to think about working with adolescents "as if" they were a group I know little about. Through reflecting on our position in relation to adolescent culture, we can take our knowledge of Theraplay and create attuned and individually tailored input with the intention of easing distress.

Each culture is likely to position adolescents in a particular frame of understanding. Aynsley-Green (2019) is wonderfully challenging of the English response to childhood and he includes adolescence within that term. In Britain, the common discourse about adolescence is disparaging. The "snowflake generation" is seen as incapable of managing the stresses and pressures of adult life. Alternatively, adolescents are labeled as dangerous and to be dispersed like animals. In some areas, this has led to the use of high-pitched sounds that only under-25s can perceive being used to move on groups of pupils perceived to be threatening (BBC, 2019). It appears that whether they are seen as pathetic or aggressive, the underlying adult view, perpetuated by popular media, is that adolescents are failing. As Blakemore (2018) points out, if we as a society were as judgmental of any other minority group, this would be unacceptable. However, if adolescence is socially constructed and so likely to be different in different cultures, is there any common ground within the worldwide community of practice that means I can give high-quality, global guidance about a starting point for work with adolescents?

Blakemore (2018), writing about the neuroscience of adolescence, identifies three reasons why we can say that adolescence is a specific and distinct developmental phase in human maturation. These can be summarized as:

1. behaviors that are associated with adolescence—risk-taking, heightened self-consciousness and the influence of peers—are seen in many different cultures

2. other mammal species display adolescent-type behaviors between infancy and full maturity

3. adolescent behavior is historically reported, such as the quote attributed to Socrates, "children now love luxury; they have bad manners, contempt for authority; they show disrespect for elders and love chatter in place of exercise" (Good Reads, 2019).

So, while we may need to adjust our own detailed understanding of how adolescence is constructed in our own time and place, it appears that there are specific behaviors that are likely to be common to all adolescents.

Blakemore (2018) explores adolescent behaviors of risk-taking, self-consciousness and influence of peers from the point of view of a neuroscientist. We, as therapeutic practitioners, base our work on interpersonal processes and internal perceptions. We are not researchers; we need to make sure that Blakemore's science-based stance fits with our pragmatic desire to alleviate distress through relationship. However, if in looking at adolescence from different angles we come up with the same developmental tasks, then our interventions, based on those tasks, are more likely to be robust. In this way, we can take the best from both quantitative and qualitative research to inform our practice.

There is a rich literature about the psychological tasks of adolescence to which it is difficult to do justice here. Fuller (2014) identifies some of those key thinkers as she forms a practical way of therapeutically addressing the developmental tasks of adolescence. She cites Erikson (1967), who identifies the development of identity and the resolution of role confusion as the key focus of adolescence. Seen from this psychosocial perspective, the adolescent will need to grapple with the anxieties that come with not knowing where they belong, or who they are as puberty changes their body, and as changes in cognition lead to a greater awareness of, and reflection on, the context in which they live.

If adolescents are likely to be part of your caseload, deepening your understanding of and sensitivity to the nuances of these development processes is a very important part of your professional development as a Theraplay practitioner. However, for the purposes of this chapter, we can focus our thinking around the areas Fuller (2014) identifies as critical to address in adolescent development. These can be summarized as:

- working with strong emotions
- encouraging communication with peers
- encouraging communication with parents
- working with the conflicting senses of wanting to be seen and not seen.

Three of these match developmental tasks that Blackmore identifies in her writing: strong emotions linking with the potential for risk-taking, issues of wanting to be seen and not seen linking with self-consciousness and, finally, how peer relationships are formed. The difference between these two authors is around the role of parents in this developmental phase. I agree with Fuller (2014) that, although there is a drive to form an independent identity in adolescence, this needs to be forged through a changing relationship with parents rather than parents no longer featuring in the adolescent's life. Parents can still be a secure base, something that is pertinent to our work as attachment-focused Theraplay practitioners.

We will now explore these four areas in relation to Theraplay practice with adolescents.

Working with strong emotions

Bainbridge (2009) tells us that the human brain is at its biggest during the teenage years. In adolescent development, that big brain, developed during childhood, has to be pruned and shaped for adulthood. As he says, a big brain is no good unless it is organized. Just as in infancy, the environment is critical to this. During this maelstrom of synaptic pruning, the experiences of the adolescent influence which synaptic connections are kept and which are lost.

The parietal cortex, an area of the brain involved in processing sensory experience, is shaped, enabling complex sensory-affective connections to be made. The prefrontal cortex, the part of the brain that helps us plan what we want and how to get it, is also significantly pruned. While this process is happening it can be harder to plan ahead, regulate emotions, consider the needs of others and restrain one's impulses (Bainbridge, 2009). At the same time, other areas of the brain are undergoing myelination. Bainbridge calls this "the equivalent of replacing the pony express with fibre-optic cable" (2009, p.108). Messages can now be transmitted faster and further in the brain. The areas that experience this myelination that Bainbridge identifies are language areas, areas linking memory and emotion, and nerve fibers that carry information from brain to muscle to support movement. That might explain the mouthy, smart, energetic, over-emotional and know-it-all adolescent who won't let you forget what you said last Monday at 2.30 precisely, then!

Bainbridge (2009) points out that while these changes may be observable via functional MRI scanning, we can't say there is a direct causal link between them and adolescent behavior. We also need to keep in mind that this is a fast-moving field and he was writing in 2009. However, I think it is safe to say that there is a lot going on in the adolescent brain that is probably going to impact how they behave in the world. Take this with the frequent negative social constructs placed on adolescence and it isn't surprising that this stage of development is confusing, painful and disorientating for both the adolescent and those who care about them.

Compare these behaviors of normal development in adolescence to symptoms of complex post-traumatic stress disorder (PTSD) as listed by the National Health Service (2019): feelings of shame or guilt, difficulty controlling your emotions, periods of losing attention and concentration, physical symptoms, such as headaches, dizziness, chest pains and stomach aches, cutting yourself off from friends and family, relationship difficulties, destructive or risky behavior, including self-harm and substance misuse, and suicidal thoughts.

Blakemore says:

> The adolescent brain isn't a dysfunctional or a defective adult brain. Adolescence is a formative period of life, when neural pathways are malleable, and passion and creativity run high. The changes that take place in the brain during this period offer us a lens through which we can begin to see ourselves anew. (2018, p.7)

Strong feelings are normal in adolescence, a needed and necessary part of a healthy process.

In the face of such intensity it can be helpful to hold the Theraplay model as a guide of "how to be," rather than "what to do." Think *structure*. What does *structure* help us feel? Regulated from the outside, so we have a sense of safety and so feel organized. If we feel contained by structure we can contain these strong emotions. We can give ourselves structure by educating ourselves about adolescence and offering psychoeducation to both parents and the adolescent themselves. We can de-pathologize the developmental process by the way we are fascinated, curious and delighted in the day-to-day, moment-to-moment ups and downs of adolescence. By this we can show there is no need to be afraid. It is a process. It will pass. This way we can prevent the ordinary trials of adolescence moving from something that sounds like complex trauma from becoming a real live trauma.

The current Theraplay literature contains very little that gives voice to the experience of people receiving Theraplay, although every practitioner has their practice-based evidence in the stories of their work. There was insufficient time in the development of this chapter to systematically gather views of adolescents about the experience and effectiveness of Theraplay to manage their strong emotions, so while this next piece of feedback is not rigorous research, it is the live voice of someone who has experienced Theraplay through childhood and adolescence via their mother—the mother being me.

 Having grown up with a "Theraplay mother" who made good use of her arsenal of Theraplay games throughout my childhood, continuing to connect with her through Theraplay into my adolescence came naturally. It helped me to find my silliness when outside pressures told me that I was supposed to be a serious young adult with serious responsibilities, and it was nice to just be a child sometimes! It also affirmed that Mum would always be there for me, to play but also to support me when things were tough, so I knew that the loving, supportive core of our relationship would always be there even though other elements of our relationship were shifting as I grew up and struck out on my own. Being the one to initiate games such as pop cheeks was also nice and it felt as if it showed Mum that even though I was becoming independent and wanted to be seen as an adult, I could still be open to playing and being cared for—that I could still be her child even if I wasn't a child anymore! I also found myself beginning to connect with my friends through Theraplay too. For example, one of my closest friends loves beep and honk! I introduced her to it when she spontaneously "booped" my nose and now she always "honks" my chin and finds it hilarious! It's nice to know that I can continue being silly as an adult in my other relationships, not just with Mum, and playing Theraplay games as an adolescent helped me to realize that.

Practitioners in training often say they are concerned that Theraplay will seem too silly or infantile to adolescents. In my experience, once adolescents have an experience of Theraplay, they lap it up. They may ask for it in a tangential way and you may get the feeling they are going along with things just to humor you, but that's fine. If they are getting multisensory, affect-attuned, attachment-supporting experience, it is good. One of the key skills in managing resistance in adolescent work is to just keep going, to be confident and to enjoy the adolescents getting the better of you in a humorous way. The biggest fears of engaging the strong emotions of adolescence via Theraplay may be our own.

Encouraging communication with peers

Working with adolescents in peer groups would seem an ideal way to use Theraplay to negotiate the key task of forging new identities by safely moving away from the identity formed within their family.

For those adolescents where we worry that they are vulnerable and might be swept into a culture that is not in their best interests, it still seems important to give them fun experiences of peer groups that will reinforce cultural "norms" that we would like them to internalize. The cultural identity created by adolescents themselves means that we need to be rigorous in our self-reflexivity about our own cultural positioning. There is a power shift from the "older, wiser and kind" position adopted with the infant and young child. We don't abdicate our wisdom, we hold very tightly to our kindness and age, but allow the adolescent to teach us a thing or two as well. We show this by how we allow the adolescent to suggest ideas for developing games and activities and negotiate with them and sometimes let them lead. This is a key adaptation of Theraplay for this developmental stage.

Blakemore (2018) identifies neurobiological changes that show that even within "adolescence" there are stages during which the adolescent will be open to different things. Younger adolescents, for example, tend to be generous with all "friends," while older adolescents are more generous towards those they see as closer to them. The older the adolescent, the more likely they are to be able to take into account the intention of someone wanting a relationship with them and are more likely to reject an offer if they perceive it to be unfair.

The younger adolescent is likely to be more generously open to including everyone put in the group. A Theraplay group aimed at helping young adolescents feel connected to each other could contain a wider spread of presenting difficulties and styles of interaction while still facilitating a general shift towards a helpful group culture.

 A teacher of early adolescent pupils approached me saying their class was getting very fractious and agitated with each other. Exams were approaching and the class teacher felt that the group as a whole was not managing the pressure very well. I theorized that this group of young adolescents had an insufficient sense of safety in the face of challenge for their maturing systems to self-regulate when faced with strong emotions stirred by formal academic testing. I felt the adolescents needed to have an experience of mastery of tension using the dimension of *challenge*. Activities from the dimensions of *structure* and *nurture* would support the process of self-regulation.

Everyone participated in some mildly challenging but structurally engaging activities. Pass the cup in rhythm was particularly popular, with the whole class developing a strong sense of togetherness as they "tap, tap, passed" paper cups around the circle. A game of matching the various ways I said "fish" to the way they said "chips" helped everyone know that the whole group could come back together after excitement. Everyone did a paper punch in groups of three, two holding the paper edges while the third punched. The whole group waited until I shouted "1-2-3 punch" to ensure that there were no accidents. On the surface, the impression was one of chaos but the activities were very highly planned and structured.

When everyone had done paper punch they all were instructed to screw the paper up into balls and the class was divided into two. A game of paper ball fight followed allowing the energy level in the room to rise to a very high level. I had anticipated this and had a whistle to use to be loud enough when the time was up. The balls on each team were counted by an adult holding open a big plastic sack for the pupils to toss the balls into, making for a quick and fun way to tidy the room. The pupils were then immediately led through a lying down mindfulness body scan exercise. This was a way to enable some nurture to be offered when there was a large number of pupils and a few adults. Overall, the session lasted 30 minutes and took the pupils through an experience of very heightened emotional states but also giving them an experience of how they could self-regulate through the mindfulness practice.

Older adolescents are more likely to approach a group with a degree of suspicion, requiring the practitioner to present the group purpose and aims with great congruence and warmth. We may, therefore, need to spend more time selecting group members and forming strong relationships with individuals within the group. If group members don't already know each other, we need to help them buy into the group aims before the group meets.

The powerful experience of feeling very alone while needing to be part of a group to face the challenges of life was brought home to me when, at a Theraplay training, I was asked whether Theraplay could be used to support a group of older adolescents where one of the peer group had a life-limiting condition. The group didn't know when their friend would die and the young person could no longer attend school but was still active on social media. The ill student was very open with peers about their condition.

Unsurprisingly, there was a range of responses in the adolescent peer group from ignoring the situation to overt and overwhelming feelings of despair and loss. Together the Theraplay trainees and I thought about the developmental tasks being faced. These peers were being faced, in a stark way, with the reality of the existential questions of "Who am I?" and "What am I here for?" Their attachment to a peer, so important in adolescence, was going to be ruptured. We felt that in this highly charged situation the peer group needed a way to connect with each other. They didn't need adults to "get them to talk about" the loss but to help them create a safe space in which they could face their feelings and support each other. A carefully designed group would support the normal adolescent process of identifying with peers to help them all manage the emotional challenge they were facing. We felt that it would be important to first provide some structure followed by engagement and nurture. Challenge would also be really important for this group to have the felt experience of mastering tensions. We theorized that by giving the group playful opportunities to "rehearse" rupture, repair and mastering tension they would have a felt experience of coping together. They would then be able to draw on this when their peer died. We also knew that any activities would need to be age appropriate for older adolescents.

We drew up the following group plan:

Goals for the group
1. To be able to accept and give nurture. To promote a sense of being able to give and receive support.
2. To create a sense of "togetherness" and safety in the face of an out-of-control event (engagement).
3. To increase the ability to tolerate uncertainty (structure and challenge).
4. To support the communication of emotional needs (nurture and structure).
Group purpose
The group needs to know why it is meeting; for example, "We all know x is really ill and we don't know what is going to happen. We know they can't be in school. This is a time where we can just be together, do stuff, and if we want to talk about x then that is fine. It's your group, I'm here to make sure there are no hurts, that you can all stick together and maybe you can have a bit of okay time. I've got some stuff to get us started today and we can see how things go…"
I wouldn't use the "have fun" rule in this circumstance. Make sure you create clear group boundaries of time; for example, "We can meet each week for the rest of this academic year and then we can think together about next year."
Activity: Parachute games
Dimensions: Structure and engagement.
How to do it: Run under the chute if you share a similarity with someone, for example shoe size, hairstyle.
Progression over time: Move to group members naming things. Start to approach the trauma and feelings that go with it.
Equipment: Parachute or sizable blanket.
Activity: Check-ins
Dimensions: Nurture, engagement with extra structure to start with.
How to do it: Compliment each person initially verbally (hairstyle, eye color, etc.).
Progression over time: Count knuckles using lotion dots in pairs and then rub in. Move towards "classic check-ins" in pairs. At some point, leader to verbalize that some hurts are not visible but still there.
Equipment: Lotion and cotton wool balls in the future.

Activity: Trust games—the in/out challenge
Dimensions: Challenge and structure.
How to do it: Stand in circle alternately facing in and out. Link arms and lean the direction you are facing. Everyone is supporting each other.
Progression over time: Increase the level of trust needed, for example shutting eyes, having to tune in to see who in the group starts the leaning rather than using verbal direction.
Equipment: None.

Activity: Foot balloon keepy uppies
Dimensions: Challenge, up-regulating but with grounding.
How to do it: Everyone lying on the floor in a circle, keeping a balloon in the air just using the feet.
Progression over time: Other cooperative challenge games.
Equipment: Balloon, maybe gym mats if the floor is hard.

Activity: Worry popcorn
Dimensions: Structure and nurture.
How to do it: Everyone takes as many cotton wool balls as they would like to represent things they have on their mind for the week ahead. Follow usual popcorn game instructions. Could progress to cotton ball fight if further release of emotion is needed.
Progression over time: In time, people can choose to name those worries or not. Be aware of possible out-of-group follow-up if needed. Watch to ensure there is cathartic release as cotton balls go flying, be aware of noise levels. Are these indicating relaxed breathing/change in muscular tensions?
Equipment: Cotton wool balls, blanket.

Activity: Group weather report
Dimensions: Nurture.
How to do it: In a circle on each other's backs.
Progression over time: A metaphorical story could be developed to share the trauma while giving privacy to each person's own response.
Equipment: None.

Activity: Closing rituals
Dimensions: Nurture, Structure, Engagement Text.
Nurture: Eat a meal together. Great if the school can provide this; if not, get people to bring a packed meal but leader to provide a treat for everyone and make sure they give it out individually.
Closing ritual: Develop with the group and with time. It may initially be a group handshake/hug/code word/song. A song doesn't have to be sung; the group might select something to play on someone's phone. The group may need to be structured initially. In time, they may choose a significant song.

As with any Theraplay intervention, the art lies in the ability to identify achievable goals for the session taking into account the presenting issues of the people you are working with.

Encouraging communication with parents

Working in Theraplay with adolescents and their parents may, on the surface, appear contradictory to the developmental drive for the adolescent to be independent. However, across the lifespan, secure attachments underpin sustained mental health and positive internal working models. One of the challenges of working with families containing adolescents is to make "securing the base" palatable despite the changing family dynamics. Even for people who have had good enough attachment relationships in their early childhoods, a secure base can be "wobbled" by life events. The developmental drives of adolescence can then seem to create blockages to the support that each family member might give each other. If the usual processes of reflective, empathetic, responsive attunement break down under stress, there is a strong possibility of each family member taking a role and getting "stuck" in it.

 Sue had three children, Mark (17), Ben (14) and Amy (12). It was a year since her husband, the children's father, had died suddenly. As a family, they had been immensely shocked. They had weathered the first year of anniversaries, but Sue was now worried about Ben who was shutting himself in his room. He was rude and aggressive towards her when she tried to ban him from having his phone in his room at night. Mark had tried to intervene, and Ben had hit him.

In these circumstances, the intention of Theraplay is not to address the trauma that the family has faced but to free up the natural healing capacities of each family member by "doing" communication rather than talking about it. This attention to the multisensory and non-verbal aspects of family dynamics can "kick start" the healthy patterns of relationship that a family have but which may have been overwhelmed, temporarily, by a high level of arousal resulting from stress and trauma.

 Sue had been very tearful in the intake meeting and somewhat surprised when the practitioner said that it sounded as if they were all doing really well and she would like to see the whole family together. Sue had expected Ben to be seen on his own. From the intake interview, the practitioner formulated the idea that each family member, as well as the family as a whole, needed to find a new identity in the face of the unexpected loss of a significant attachment figure. Ben was particularly struggling as developmentally he needed to withdraw, while at the same time he needed the support of his family to manage the loss of his dad.

When the family arrived for their first session, Ben was very flat, Mark very serious and Amy tried to be the life and soul of the family. Sue just looked bewildered as the practitioner got the family to bat a balloon to each other. It was clear from this engaging game that Ben was struggling to manage the connection to his family. It was as if Amy was sucking up all the family energy to make herself so visible that they were distracted from grief. She seemed to want to force Ben to play while Mark alternatively cajoled Ben or tried to squash Amy's exuberance. The pain in the room was palpable, but to find ways to talk about the loss felt too unsafe while the family communication seemed so stuck. Structure was needed to create a sense of external regulation, along with engagement to help each family member find a level of arousal that allowed a shared sense of connection.

The practitioner moved from balloon keepy uppies to inviting each family member to make a body shape for the other to copy. The practitioner used Group Theraplay thinking to show she was in charge; she indicated when it was each family member's turn and, in a firm and compassionate way, she prevented Amy from stepping in and making disparaging comments when it was Ben's turn. Ben showed how overwhelmed he felt in his slumped body. Mark and Sue copied. Amy resisted.

Slowly, Ben became more involved. As the session progressed and the balance shifted from structure activities to engagement, he started to find his "voice." In a game of "what's the weirdest noise you can make?" he put his hand under his armpit and made a loud farting noise, looking embarrassed and then relieved when his mother and brother fell about laughing.

Sue emailed the practitioner after the session. When they got home, Ben put the television on in the lounge, something he hadn't done for months. Amy went to her room. Later, Sue heard her crying. It was the first time she had cried since her dad had died. Sue went and sat on her bed and stroked her head. Ben brought them both a cup of tea, looking rather sheepish as he spilled it putting it down. When Sue said "Thank you" she was able to have full eye contact with him. Sue said that that was when she knew it was going to be all right and when she realized just how much she had missed Ben over the past year.

Using a Group Theraplay approach works well with families where there have been good enough attachments that have been disrupted by life events such as the family described above. However, this approach may not be suitable for families where there are underlying attachment difficulties manifesting as children with significantly avoidant or ambivalent attachment styles, or those nearing disorganization. Such attachment patterns may have positive adaptive elements that have protected children within the family dynamic. However, families that have just about been coping may be tipped into not coping once adolescence is manifest by children listening to peers more than adults, taking risks and having little motivation to see another person's point of view. This may manifest as the onset of mental health difficulty in the adolescent.

The outcome of all therapy is dependent on the quality of the relationship developed between the client and the therapist (Wampold, 2015). Fuller and Smart (2016) affirm that the quality of the relationship is vital to the young person investing in the therapeutic process. Where family relationships have broken down it may initially be inappropriate to have everyone in the same room at the same time—although that is clearly what we would want to be working towards as Theraplay practitioners. First, however, we may need to form strong relationships with each family member. The roots of adolescent distress may well lie in the mental health status of the parents, in which case, just as we would with younger children, we would need to invest time in working with the parents. However, because of the adolescent potential for risk-taking behaviors, we may need to actively engage the adolescent at the same time. Having a team to work with is really helpful, but if you are a sole practitioner it is essential that you set out the limits of confidentiality, identify goals for the work, and make sure that everyone can sign up to give enough time to the case.

The majority of parents want the best for their children and want to protect them from harm or hardship. What worked when the children were tiny no longer works with the adolescent as the drive to connect is now away from the primary caregiving relationship. The adolescent brain also needs sleep at a different time from the rest of the family. The adolescent body is driven to express itself in different ways, with lumps and bumps appearing unbidden and sometimes unwanted and things all feeling rather out of control. The logical step of an anxious parent is to try to take back control, but now that drives a wedge into the relationship.

As a Theraplay practitioner you are there to support the "No Hurts" rule, and that means facilitating the sharing of appropriate power and enabling parents to mourn the loss of the relationship they once had with their child while celebrating the arrival of a developing adult who needs non-possessive support and guidance to emerge into the world.

Our first step with all family members, therefore, may be psycho-education. I want the parent to be as fascinated and captivated by the amazing dynamics of the adolescent brain as I am. That warm fascination and non-judgmental amazement at the person before us can be the foundation from which a new relationship with an emerging adult can be formed.

More so than when working with many other ages and stages of development, with families containing adolescents with avoidant or ambivalent-type attachments, Theraplay becomes a way of thinking about what is needed, a framework for making sense of the complex information that comes your way in families coming for help. Huge levels of flexibility are required. In the same session, with the same individual, you may have to support three-year-old developmental needs as the adolescent regresses (using some really young Theraplay games such as beep and honk) as well as adult-to-adult relationships when the young person is in that mode (which may involve more complex challenge-based games). You may need to facilitate actual talking about shifting non-verbal and somatic learning into thinking about and reflecting on family experiences and issues. Integrating modalities such as dyadic developmental psychotherapy (Hughes, 2011) or other verbal family-based ways of working may be required.

In many ways, the fluidity of the developmental process and the rapidity of the young person flitting between emotional ages is very reminiscent of working with children with relational trauma. A good history, taken with parents and checked out with the adolescent, will help you identify the core attachment representations that people are bringing into the work to make sure you don't confuse "ordinary adolescence" with disorganized attachment. The MIM is a powerful way to see, hear and experience the attachment patterns of the family in action. Undertaking a MIM as your first interaction with adolescents and their families can be helpful. For the first time, the young person who may have been labeled as the "problem" suddenly finds the focus isn't about them or what they might be doing to themselves, but on the family as a whole. Clearly you need to make a judgment about the emotional fragility of the young person, but I would also consider doing a MIM feedback for the adolescent on their own as well as for the parents. This can be really useful in forming a relationship of trust with the young person.

Working with the conflicting senses of wanting to be seen and not seen

Blakemore tells us that "Cognitive processes that rely on the prefrontal cortex, including many executive functions such as the ability to inhibit automatic behavior, undergo substantial and protracted development in adolescence" (2018, p.90). Adults with damage to this brain area find it difficult to change behavior that could be seen as rude, socially inappropriate or impulsive. They may be emotionally reactive. With this part of the adolescent brain still being under construction, it is not surprising that similar behavior is part of their repertoire.

Many of the impulsive, risk-taking behaviors of adolescence result in mild inconvenience and are a rich source of embarrassing tales that can be told later in life. However, with the intensity of feeling that is present in adolescents, these experiences can tip over into shame, and with shame there is the strong need to hide away either through withdrawal or through making others withdraw by unpleasant or aggressive behaviors.

Shanice was adopted when she was nine months old. Her adoptive mother was white, her adoptive father black, and she was mixed race.

When she was three, her parents split up, with her mother going on to marry her stepfather. Her family then consisted of Shanice, her white mother, her white stepfather and his two children who were also white. From an early age, Shanice felt too visible and as if she didn't "fit." At 15, she traced her birth mother via social media. She argued with her family, drank and was defiant at school. At 16, her stepfather told her to leave the family home. She sofa surfed, eventually finding a place in a hostel. By 18 she had become a mother herself.

Somerville *et al.* (2013) found that if adolescents believed a peer was observing them then this in itself was sufficient to cause a high level of self-consciousness, higher than for either children or adults. Such self-consciousness will likely be further elevated if there is a fear of being judged and found wanting by people who they perceive to have "power over" them.

 Shanice was placed in a small bedsit with her baby. Soon social services became involved because of concern about the baby's lack of weight gain and Shanice's poor personal hygiene. Heather, a social worker who had been trained in Theraplay, was allocated the case. While doing her statutory duties it became clear to her that Shanice was not listening and was becoming more and more withdrawn, agitated and possibly aggressive. Heather initially felt angry, then helpless, something she recognized as a countertransference response. Heather discussed the visit with her Theraplay supervisor, even though it wasn't a case that had been referred for Theraplay. Together they considered how exposed Shanice might be feeling, as well as how overwhelmed by the challenges of new parenthood in such unsupportive accommodation. They felt she needed engagement to help her connect with Heather, but they thought the level of shame might get in the way of this process. Heather talked about her dual role of needing to ensure that Shanice was providing for her baby in a good enough way, which required Heather to make judgments, while wanting to be non-judgmentally supportive to Shanice.

Cairns (2004) identifies shame as an important early developmental phase in which the parent helps the toddler separate their sense of self from their behavior. Shame can then shift to guilt and becomes a tool to help modify behavior. For the adolescent processing the experience of wanting to be seen and also not be seen, shame is an overwhelming state of being "too visible." Shame felt in the raw is disabling, leading to a felt state of utter inadequacy. If our socially constructed positioning of adolescents also labels them as inadequate, then here is a risk. How easy it would have been for Shanice to have her baby removed instead of receiving support that might enable her to process this developmental stage.

A Theraplay practitioner working with adolescents may need to be both a buffer between the adult world and the adolescent, and a translator of the adolescent to the adult world to shift shame to guilt. When shame becomes guilt, there is a motivation for behavior change.

 Heather and her supervisor talked about what it might feel like to Shanice if Heather played Theraplay games with the baby to try to show Shanice how to engage. Heather role-played Shanice to help her work out what this might be like and from the role play thought this would be very difficult for Shanice, causing her to feel even more isolated and de-skilled. At their next meeting, sitting beside Shanice so there was no eye contact, Heather took a baby doll onto her lap and started to count the doll's toes and sing nursery rhymes. She could feel Shanice relaxing beside her and watching what she was doing and listening to her singsong tone. When Shanice's baby woke up, Heather observed Shanice being a little gentler. As she laid the baby on the changing mat she glanced towards Heather. Heather smiled and asked Shanice if she would like her to teach the song she had been singing. Shanice didn't answer but seemed relaxed as Heather knelt on the floor beside her. With Heather singing, Shanice slowly and kindly changed her baby's nappy.

It took many weeks and a lot of hard work by Heather to protect the emotional space she'd made with Shanice. Her managers wanted her to say whether or not the baby should be removed. Heather felt Shanice slowly starting to relax in her presence, and through the parallel play of Heather with the baby doll and Shanice playing with her own baby, the level of engagement started to grow. Shanice started accepting some degree of nurture, verbal at first but then accepting a hand massage from Heather. Heather always checked in with Shanice, making some compliments about her. The first time she tried to acknowledge a "hurt" by noticing how tired Shanice looked, Shanice took this as a criticism, so Heather said, "I am sorry, I didn't word that very well. I just meant it is very hard to find the time to rest when you are putting your baby's needs first."

Shanice started to seem brighter. She managed to get a pushchair so she could take her baby out and she told Heather about talking to the ducks in the park. Heather made up a song about "this little ducky went to market" and taught it to Shanice, who thought it was funny. It was the first time Heather had seen her smile. Shanice then sang the song to her baby. Heather took this as a sign that she could be more direct with Shanice and she started to demonstrate engaging and nurturing games directly with Shanice, saying they were so she could play them with her baby but also knowing that Shanice herself had significant unmet needs to connect with someone, feel as if she belonged and feel good about herself. Shanice developed enough trust in Heather to allow her to secure funding for more formal Theraplay.

As Shanice matured from adolescence to young adulthood, as she saw the needs of her baby and how to meet them and as she experienced the pleasure of her baby responding to her, Shanice could think about her adoptive mum and hold a more complex view because she could begin to put herself in her mother's shoes. With Heather's help, she contacted her adoptive mum. Both Shanice and her adoptive mum came to Theraplay parent feedback sessions and her adoptive mum started to understand what might have caused Shanice to feel so excruciatingly visible and at the same time invisible in the family. With the relationship between Shanice and her adoptive mother restored, Heather ended her work.

As Theraplay practitioners we may not be likely to be explicit about our belief in human nature, our "acts of faith" in the broadest sense, not necessarily connected to any specific religious or spiritual practice. However, I would argue that in working with adolescents we do put our faith in a self-actualizing principle. We water seeds that have been sown at earlier stages of development. Sometimes we know how they blossom, sometimes we don't, but we trust the human spirit that, if at all possible, things grow well.

 Heather came across Shanice a few years later when Shanice had a placement as part of her social work training. After their work had ended, Shanice had re-established contact with old school friends, developed enough trust in her mother to allow her to provide childcare for her baby, returned to college and gained the qualification to go to university to study for her social work degree. The first thing she did when she saw Heather was to pull out her phone and show her pictures of her baby who was now a smiling, healthy and robust young child enjoying the care of two generations of strong adult women.

The need to be seen/not seen in adolescence led to a decision about the stories in this chapter. Families are generous in giving consent for their stories to be shared and I take seriously the trust they place in me. However, it is usually the adults in the family who mediate that consent, although I ask that it is discussed with everyone. Keeping in mind that people may change their views about consent as they mature, or feel they can't say no at the time, the stories in this chapter (except that of my child) are fictionalized from many different cases and no one should be able to identify themselves now or in the future.

Working with the adolescent who has experienced trauma

Early in this chapter I suggested that the normal processes of development in adolescence are reminiscent of the symptoms of complex PTSD. Both the "normally" developing and the traumatized adolescent might show poor self-regulation, rejection of the social bonds that would actually lead to a felt experience of safety and a world view that is radically different from that of their primary caregivers. I suggested that as Theraplay practitioners we need to be mindful of this and not see trauma where actually there is "merely" the storm of adolescence going on.

However, some adolescents have experienced early disrupted relationships and have not been able to develop any organization of their response to their primary caregiver—that is, they have disorganized attachment styles. Although exact definitions can be debated and fine distinctions made, for the purposes of this chapter I use the terms disorganized attachment, relational trauma, complex trauma and developmental trauma interchangeably, using the general term "trauma." I am not referring to adolescents who have experienced a single incident trauma; this might be better addressed with eye movement desensitization reprocessing (EMDR) (Gomez & Jernberg, 2013), although Theraplay could still be helpful in creating a sense of safety in a family to support trauma processing.

In reviewing the literature that I commonly refer to when considering how I might adapt Theraplay for children with trauma (Damasio, 2012; Panksepp, 2005; Porges, 2011; Sieff, 2015; Struik, 2014), I was surprised that few list "adolescents" or "adolescence" in their index. The exceptions were Cozolino (2002) and Hughes (2011), both of whom mention adolescence briefly. However, all these authors talk a great deal about trauma in children.

When a child experiences relational or developmental trauma, the usual process of childhood development takes second place to the more pressing need for emotional survival. Reflecting on my own practice of Theraplay with adolescents and trying to work out what adaptations I make for trauma, I concluded that these are the same as those I make for younger children. This makes sense as one can theorize that the emotional part of their development is stuck at a much earlier stage than their chronological age. I therefore recommend you refer to Chapter 9 in the third edition of *Theraplay* (Booth & Jernberg, 2010) and the chapters on working with the traumas of child sexual abuse and domestic violence in this volume when you are considering Theraplay with adolescents who have experienced trauma.

Questions for reflection and continued learning

1. Without an understanding of typical or atypical development in adolescence, we can feel as if we are dealing with an alien species. It can be helpful to hold our cultural humility in mind when considering people identified as adolescents. How do you seek to understand your socially constructed position in relation to adolescence? How does your personal and cultural history impact your countertransference response to adolescents in Theraplay?

2. How did you have fun as an adolescent? How do you have fun now? How can you demonstrate to an adolescent that growing up is "worth it"?

3. How will you distinguish between the "normal" turmoil of adolescence and identifying adolescents who have experienced trauma?

References

Aynsley-Green, A. (2019). *The British Betrayal of Childhood: Challenging Uncomfortable Truths and Bringing About Change* (first edition). New York, NY: Routledge.

Bainbridge, D. (2009). *Teenagers: A Natural History*. London, UK: Portobello.

BBC. (2019). *Teenagers "Should Challenge Use of Mosquito Devices."* Retrieved from www.bbc.co.uk/news/uk-politics-16273076.

Blakemore, S.J. (2018). *Inventing Ourselves: The Secret Life of the Teenage Brain*. Retrieved from www.overdrive.com/search?q=FA5F1EBF-5810-4CCC-9A1C-7842D206535A.

Booth, P.B. & Jernberg, A.M. (2010). *Theraplay: Helping Parents and Children Build Better Relationships through Attachment-Based Play*. San Francisco, CA: Jossey-Bass.

Cairns, K. (2004). *Attachment, Trauma and Resilience: Therapeutic Caring for Children* (reprinted). London, UK: British Association for Adoption and Fostering.

Cozolino, L.J. (2002). *The Neuroscience of Psychotherapy: Building and Rebuilding the Human Brain*. New York, NY: W.W. Norton & Company.

Damasio, A.R. (2012). *Self Comes to Mind: Constructing the Conscious Brain*. London, UK: Vintage Books.

Erikson, E.H. (1967). *Identity, Youth and Crisis*. New York, NY: W.W. Norton & Company.

Fuller, T. (2014). "Working with the Developmental Tasks of Adolescence During the Secondary School Years." In C. McLaughlin & C. Holliday *Therapy with Children and Young People: Integrative Counselling in Schools and Other Settings* (pp.65–85). London, UK: SAGE Publications.

Fuller, T. & Smart, T. (2016). "Working in Partnership with Adolescents in Care who have Experienced Early Trauma." In M. Richardson, F. Peacock, G. Brown, T. Fuller, T. Smart & J. Williams *Fostering Good Relationships: Partnership Work in Therapy with Children Looked After and Adopted* (pp.117–132). London, UK: Karnac Books.

Gomez, A.M. & Jernberg, E. (2013). "Using EMDR Therapy and Theraplay." In A. Gomez *EMDR Therapy and Adjunct Approaches with Children* (pp.273–297). New York, NY: Springer Publishing.

Good Reads. (2019). Retrieved from www.goodreads.com/quotes/63219-the-children-now-love-luxury-they-have-bad-manners-contempt.

Hughes, D.A. (2011). *Attachment-Focused Family Therapy Workbook* (first edition). New York, NY: W.W. Norton & Company.

Krause, I.-B. (2002). *Culture and System in Family Therapy*. London, UK: Karnac.

National Health Service. (2019). Retrieved from www.nhs.uk/conditions/post-traumatic-stress-disorder-ptsd/complex.

Panksepp, J. (2005). *Affective Neuroscience: The Foundations of Human and Animal Emotions*. Oxford, UK: Oxford University Press.

Porges, S.W. (2011). *The Polyvagal Theory: Neurophysiological Foundations of Emotions, Attachment, Communication, and Self-Regulation* (first edition). New York, NY: W.W. Norton & Company.

Sieff, D.F. (ed.). (2015). *Understanding and Healing Emotional Trauma: Conversations with Pioneering Clinicians and Researchers*. London, UK; New York, NY: Routledge/Taylor & Francis.

Somerville, L.H., Jones, R.M., Ruberry, E.J., Dyke, J.P., Glover, G. & Casey, B.J. (2013). "The medial prefrontal cortex and the emergence of self-conscious emotion in adolescence." *Psychological Science, 24*(8), 1554–1562.

Struik, A. (2014). *Treating Chronically Traumatized Children: Don't Let Sleeping Dogs Lie!* London, UK; New York, NY: Routledge/Taylor & Francis.

Wampold, B.E. (2015). *The Great Psychotherapy Debate: The Evidence for What Makes Psychotherapy Work* (second edition). New York, NY: Routledge.

Chapter 5

Sunshine Circles: Universal Best Practice for Young Children in Preschool Classrooms

Kay Schieffer

Introduction

Sunshine Circles is the name we have given to our Theraplay play groups in early childhood programs. This name came about because we sang "You are My Sunshine" as our welcome activity and used a picture of a smiling sun on our visual calendar to indicate where these play groups fell in our schedule. Although the activities of Group Theraplay and Sunshine Circles are similar, we continue to distinguish Sunshine Circles because they are led by classroom teachers rather than mental health providers and the training includes special consideration of issues related to classroom practices and the mission and policies of educational institutions.

Sunshine Circles are intended to be used as universal instruction and support for social-emotional development. While Theraplay-based groups can be used with any age group, they are particularly well suited to early childhood programs. Typical early classrooms include a diverse population and require instructional strategies that are effective in groups and flexible enough to support simultaneous participation of children with a wide variety of abilities. General education classrooms include non-English speakers, children from a variety of races and ethnicities, typically developing children, children with identified disabilities and children at risk for disabilities and school failure. Teachers and staff are expected to help all these children learn to regulate their behavior and use prosocial skills such as sharing and taking turns, as well as to develop friendship skills such as asking a peer to play. Development of social skills is a universal goal of early childhood education and should be supported by matching universal strategies. Sunshine Circles are an effective and amazingly accessible instructional strategy in early childhood programs.

Key points

1. Success in school involves both social-emotional and social cognition skills because social interactions, attention and self-control affect readiness for learning (Jones, Greenberg & Crowley, 2016). Because young children are experiential learners they gain skills by doing the thing (e.g., waiting for a turn) rather than by talking about the thing. The early childhood teacher's job is to provide a wide variety of experiences that allow children to practice using the desired skill. Classroom teachers can set young children on the path to school success by providing experiences in which children actively participate in healthy social interactions that promote social-emotional functioning.

2. Sunshine Circles can help to establish a sense of emotional connection between children and their teachers. Children who feel this connection are more engaged in learning activities and have more positive social and academic outcomes. Emotional connection develops through shared joyful moments that are created in the group play. Engaging activities help children to feel individually seen and appreciated even within the group structure.

3. Sunshine Circles support attachment and regulation, which act as interrelated buffers that promote resilience. When teachers and children have an emotional connection, teachers can effectively co-regulate children to help them successfully participate in motivating activities. Teachers support the development of self-regulation by helping children control their excitement and their bodies so that they have fun in shared play.

4. Promoting attachment and regulation in the classroom is even more important for young children experiencing chronic stress

who are at greater risk for social problems and academic failure than children who do not experience chronic stress. Sunshine Circles create warm relationships and opportunities for co-regulation that are necessary to support children whose development has been impacted by adverse experiences and/or daily stressors.

5. Adult-led group play creates opportunities for children who are chronically dysregulated to acquire and practice prosocial skills. Sunshine Circles provide a bridge back into the group for children who might otherwise be excluded from peer play and have fewer opportunities to develop social skills. The adult structure and co-regulation in Sunshine Circles ensure that children can play together successfully so that everyone gets a chance to grow.

Theoretical foundations

Sunshine Circles are a type of Theraplay delivered in a group format. They are designed to provide children with a positive, well-regulated, emotionally rich and rewarding experience with other children and trustworthy adults. Through play, the teacher creates sequences of interpersonal connection and care with the child, using the model of a healthy parent-child relationship. The model's unique combination of social engagement, interpersonal play and nurture expands the child's window of tolerance for stress while helping the child to practice healthy social-emotional skills.

Along with other varieties of Theraplay, Sunshine Circles are based on four dimensions of healthy parent-child interaction: *structure*, *engagement*, *nurture* and *challenge*. These dimensions are embedded into four rules used for conveying the intent of the interactions in a playful and accessible way. Those rules are: No Hurts (nurture), Stick Together (engagement), Have Fun (playful challenge) and the Adult is in Charge (structure). Each Sunshine Circle session repeats the same sequence of activities: Welcome, Check-In, Games, Food Share and Goodbye activity. All of these elements taken together allow the child to feel safe at a deep, brain-stem level well below the level of consciousness. This felt safety becomes the essential foundation for the child's participation and success in school.

Children's level of social and emotional functioning is widely recognized as an indicator of the development of executive functioning and school readiness (Blair, 2003; Blair & Raver, 2012, Raver, 2004). Social-emotional functioning is so essential to student outcomes that some states have proposed that outcomes be assessed using a set of standards similar to those for academic achievement (McClelland & Tominey, 2014). Children who are motivated and connected to others in the early years of schooling are much more likely to establish positive trajectories of development in both social and academic domains (Baker, Grant & Morlock, 2008; Hamre & Pianta, 2007; Silver *et al.*, 2005;). Teachers' abilities to support social and emotional functioning in the classroom are therefore central to any model of effective classroom practice. Research continues to confirm that early intervention for social-emotional needs has a greater impact on outcomes than does later remediation (Baker *et al.*, 2008; Jones, Greenberg & Crowley, 2016).

Developmental theory and research suggest that interactions between children and adults are the primary mechanism of child development and learning (Hamre & Pianta, 2007; Mashburn *et al.*, 2008). Large-scale classroom observation studies in the National Institute of Child Health and Human Development concluded that, in early childhood programs, child-adult interactions are more influential on outcomes than the presence of materials, physical environment or specific curriculum (National Institute of Child Health and Human Development Early Care Research Network, 2002; National Scientific Council on the Developing Child, 2015). Predictors of student performance on standardized literacy tests in preschool and first grade include teacher awareness of children's learning and emotional concerns, and the emotional connection, respect and enjoyment demonstrated between teachers and children and among children (Hamre & Pianta, 2005; National Institute of Child Health and Human Development Early Care Research Network, 2003). Studies show that children who are able to form secure attachments to their teachers have higher levels of engagement in learning activities and higher scores in literacy and math assessments (Geddes, 2006).

A large body of research confirms that emotional connections with caregivers and teachers also promote improved resilience and self-esteem in young children. There is a growing consensus that increasing caregiver attunement and responsiveness are important aspects of early social and emotional intervention for building resilience (Asok *et al.*, 2013). Researchers have emphasized the importance of caregivers such as daycare providers and teachers as well as parents in promoting resilience in children (Masten, 2013; Masten *et al.*, 2008). Research suggests that the development of stable child-caregiver (parent, teacher, childcare provider) attachment occurs in conjunction with the development of regulatory skills in young children experiencing adversity. The secure relationship provides a protective buffer through the co-regulation provided within the relationship. The active teaching of skills related to executive functioning and self-regulation provides young children with resources to draw on during stressful moments (Masten *et al.*, 2008; National Scientific Council on the Developing Child, 2015). These factors may provide a child with access to both co-regulation with a caregiver (i.e., "Let's take a break and we'll calm down") and self-regulation through the learned strategies (i.e., "I remember to take a break to be calm") when facing stressful challenges.

For children at risk for school failure, effective early support for social-emotional development is critical. A large body of research has documented the increased risk for social difficulties and academic failure for children from minority populations and children who are chronically exposed to stress. The impact of toxic stress is seen across all developmental domains and leads to significant changes in the development of cognitive and self-regulatory capacity in young children (Kertes *et al.*, 2016; Luby *et al.*, 2013; Oh *et al.*, 2018). These changes in development can impair later development of healthy emotional regulation and resilience even when stress is no longer considered to be at toxic levels (Loman & Gunnar, 2010; Shonkoff, Boyce & McEwen, 2009). Children experiencing chronic stressors who do not receive well-matched co-regulation from an adult may develop patterns of chronic dysregulation which prevent joyful engagement and reciprocal social interactions (Lieberman *et al.*, 2011; Lillas & Turnbull, 2009).

When families live in conditions of chronic stress, children and their caregivers often have fewer opportunities for shared joy, play, stimulation, exploration and growth (Lillas & Turnbull, 2009). Fewer opportunities for shared play also result in fewer opportunities to have "serve and return" interactions that are the mechanism for creating the architecture of the right-brain neurobiological systems critical to emotional processing and stress regulation (Facompre, Bernard & Waters, 2018; Schore, 2000; Schore & Schore, 2008).

The development of self-regulation is a major developmental milestone. Learning to manage attention and emotions well enough to complete tasks, organize behavior, inhibit impulses and solve problems is challenging for all young children and especially so for those who have added developmental challenges resulting from experiencing chronic stress (McClelland & Tominey, 2014; Murray *et al.*, 2015). When children struggle with self-regulation it is even harder for them to practice prosocial skills because of the difficulty with participating in shared activities. The child who becomes too upset too easily, knocks down blocks too quickly or pushes others aside in his excitement to be first in line is often excluded by peers. Effective co-regulation in the classroom requires the teachers to give warm and responsive interactions that provide the support, coaching and modeling that children need to "understand, express, and modulate their thoughts, feelings and behaviors" (McClelland & Tominey, 2014, p.8; see also Murray *et al.*, 2015).

Effective co-regulation by teachers requires the adults to attune to children well enough to read their cues and respond consistently and sensitively with just the right amount of support. Co-regulated group play creates the opportunity for children to practice social skills with peers in a way that maximizes connectedness and minimizes "acting-out" behaviors. Repeated experiences with effective co-regulated peer play develop a capacity for the self-regulation that underpins academic and social success through adulthood (Raby *et al.*, 2015).

Effectiveness of Sunshine Circles in preschool classrooms

Two studies indicate the effectiveness of Sunshine Circles as instructional support for social-emotional development. The first randomized trial in Head Start classrooms with 206 students demonstrated significant improvements in social-emotional skills, behavior regulation, problem solving and fine motor development in the group receiving Sunshine Circles intervention (Tucker *et al.*, 2017). A classroom quality measure also indicated significant improvement in teacher sensitivity and positive regard for their students. Based on these findings, Sunshine Circles demonstrate promise as a group-based intervention that can be embedded within early childhood education curricula.

A second study tested the effects of Sunshine Circles in a two-phase randomized trial involving 189 preschool students attending Head Start preschool. Classrooms were randomly assigned to either a Sunshine Circles intervention group or a waitlist control group. In phase two, the intervention group continued with Sunshine Circles intervention, and Sunshine Circles intervention was introduced to the control participants. All of the classrooms used curricula approved by the Head Start program. Preschoolers were compared, using standardized measures of social-emotional functioning collected at three points throughout the study period. (This study will be submitted for publication in the future.)

Quantitative results indicated that Sunshine Circles, when used regularly in early childhood group settings, may lead to improved social and emotional development in areas such as attachment, self-regulation, making friends, solving problems and taking the initiative.

Results of the study also indicated that positive gains can be made in related developmental areas such as communication. They also indicated a steep decrease in problem behaviors for the treatment group. Overall, data indicated gains across a range of measures for children receiving intervention the entire year, and gains for the waitlist group once the intervention began. Findings indicate that steeper growth may be expected in the first half of the school year due to initial adjustments to school, indicating that it may be particularly important to begin the school year with the classroom bonding and connection facilitated by Sunshine Circles. Findings suggest Sunshine Circles is an effective way to reduce problem behavior and increase prosocial behavior in early childhood settings—a universal goal of preschool and early prevention programs.

When children receive early support to develop positive relationships with peers and adults, such as that provided in Sunshine Circles, there may be cascading effects for a child's developmental trajectory. Given the impact of Sunshine Circles on important proxy measures of child well-being and feelings of safety, it appears to help a class build bonds, relax with one another and spend more time in positive states, exploration and growth—experiences cited by Greenspan (2007) as important for a happy, healthy life.

CASE ILLUSTRATION

The Head Start preschool classroom was located at the end of a long hallway in an elementary school in the Midwest. The school was established in a neighborhood considered to be at-risk because of the predominance of low-income housing. The neighborhood included a large number of immigrant families, many of whom had been resettled after living for years in refugee camps. As a result, the classroom of 20 four-year-olds included children from North and Central Africa, Central America and East Asia. Four children in the classroom were English speakers. One child was in foster care, one had a diagnosis of autism, one of ADHD, and one was living with his mother and siblings in a shelter for victims of domestic violence. During the year, two highly mobile families had their students attend three different schools. All of the children were living in poverty, a condition of eligibility for the Head Start program. This mix of students was typical for classrooms in this school.

It was my third year working with this teacher and a teaching assistant as the assigned consultant for the program. The teacher and assistant had incorporated Sunshine Circles into their social-emotional curriculum after participating in a district-wide training several years before. We had planned together to start Sunshine Circles the first week of the school and to include it in the schedule for at least one "morning meeting" time every week during the school year. We made Sunshine Circles plans for the first four weeks of school knowing that I would participate as an additional supporting adult. From our previous experience, we predicted that after four sessions the children would have learned the Sunshine Circles routines and we would then reassess whether or not my help was still needed. As it turned out, the class was not well settled into the routines of Sunshine Circles until week six when I was able to fade from weekly attendance without disrupting the group.

During the first days of school there were equal parts tears and wild excitement from the children. Many were being separated from parents for the first time and left in an environment with strangers who did not speak their language. Some children zoomed around the room pulling all toys and materials off the shelf, then moving on to the next shelf without actually playing with the objects. A few children found a sheltered place to stand in the room and remained very still looking a little shell-shocked. Many children did not appear to have play schemes. A few engaged in parallel play but no children interacted in play, and some appeared unaware that there were any others in the room.

The teacher and a teaching assistant had been a team for several years and knew that their first job was to help these children form a community in which they could play together and move through daily routines as a group. Getting children to interact is critical in preschool because children can only learn some of the most important skills in interactions and shared activities. For example, the only instruction for the English language in preschool is communication during interactions; in other words, the only way that these preschoolers were going to learn English was by playing with adults and peers. The Sunshine Circles intervention was chosen deliberately to accelerate the process of forming community and stimulating interaction.

EARLY WEEKS

Our plan was to teach the sequence of activities and help everyone learn names during the first four Sunshine Circles. Our plan for each session relied heavily on the use of music and rhythm and required no individual "performance" from the children. We gathered the children for Sunshine Circle by singing and clapping "Come to Circle, Come to Circle, it is time to play" to the tune of *Frere Jacques* while walking through the room. Adults sang the Sunshine Song as the Welcome activity. For Check-In, the adults sang a simple rhythmic "hello" song using each child's name and waving a hand. During the first months of the school year, the first activity of every session was also a song with big gestures such as *Cuddly Koalas* or *Wheels on the Bus*. For Food Share, teachers first rubbed hand sanitizer on each child's hands, intentionally using the opportunity to make eye contact and connect and then gave each child a small paper cup with several crackers in it. The Goodbye was another song using children's names. The transition out of the Circle was a game. The teacher held up a colored card saying "If you are wearing red you can go to the…" while the assistant physically guided the children out of the group.

In the early weeks of our Sunshine Circles we used rather minimal direct nurturing touch compared to the amount of touch we used in sessions later in the year. This decision was based on our assessment that rubbing in lotion or feeding was too intense for most of the children while they were still adjusting to separation from parents and were just getting to know us. We believed that our best strategy for successfully introducing Sunshine Circles as an emotionally safe, predictable and joyful time was to use high levels of rhythm and structure to keep everyone together while moving rather quickly between a few activities.

THE NEXT 30 WEEKS

After four weeks of participating in Sunshine Circles once a week, every child in the class could independently follow the routine. Some very active or more withdrawn children continued to need individual assistance, but they knew what to do even if they needed help doing it. Over the next 30 weeks of the school year, the Sunshine Circles relied less and less on rhythm to keep the group together. I continued to participate through week six when most of the children could join in independently. After that time, I participated in the playgroup once a month through to the end of the school year. In week five, the Check-In and Food Share were changed to be more directly nurturing. Check-In was changed to putting lotion on hands, and Food Share was changed to placing a single cracker either in the child's mouth or in their hand. A variety of games were introduced, and the structure of games was changed to include whole group, partner and individual activities. More challenge games were introduced, with newspaper bust and bean-bag tossing games being among the favorites. One very noticeable difference by week five was the noise level during the group. Early groups were very quiet, but groups grew quite noisy as children became more emotionally comfortable. During Check-In and Food Share, children were talking to the adults and with each other. During games there were shouts, laughter and clapping. As children grew in their ability to self-regulate, we increased the use of more up-regulating games such as Duck, Duck, Goose and parachute games. Mirroring games and modulating activities were used to down-regulate children to a quieter state before they could transition out of the group.

FINAL WEEKS

During the final weeks of school, we planned Sunshine Circles to include a combination of "greatest hits" and prepared to say goodbye. Polls were taken and favorite games were played again. Favorite snacks were served again, with acknowledgment of who liked what best. During the final weeks, every group included nurturing activities such as lotion handprints and finding shapes in hands. Children were measured with a variety of materials to celebrate how they had grown. During the final group, the children worked together to make a rainbow of all of their handprints on a large banner. The Sunshine Circles became a real celebration of their evolution from anxious preschoolers to confident kindergarten-ready preschoolers!

Conclusion

Sunshine Circles provide effective universal classroom support for the development of social skills and self-regulation in young children. The Circles promote the attachment and regulation that are buffers against the effects of chronic stress and help children become more resilient. As children are motivated and able to fully participate in social activities, they are also developing executive functioning skills and are more likely to remain engaged in learning activities which lead to improved academic outcomes.

Questions for reflection and continued learning

1. What is the relationship between child-teacher attachment and development of self-regulation and resilience in young children?

2. How do Sunshine Circles support development of classroom community?

3. Why would Sunshine Circles be considered universal support?

References

Asok, A., Bernard, K., Roth, T.L., Rosen, J.B. & Dozier, M. (2013). "Parental responsiveness moderates the association between early-life stress and reduced telomere length." *Development and Psychopathology, 25*(3), 577–585.

Baker, J.A., Grant, S. & Morlock, L. (2008). "The teacher-student relationship as a developmental context for children with internalizing or externalizing behavior problems." *School Psychology Quarterly, 23*, 3–15.

Blair, C. (2003). "Behavioral inhibition and behavioral activation in young children: Relations with self-regulation and adaptation to preschool in children attending Head Start." *Developmental Psychobiology, 42*(3), 301–311.

Blair, C. & Raver, C.C. (2012). "Child development in the context of adversity: Experiential canalization of brain and behavior." *American Psychologist, 67*(4), 309–318.

Facompre, C.R., Bernard, K. & Waters, T.E.A. (2018). "Effectiveness of interventions in preventing disorganized attachment: A meta-analysis." *Development and Psychopathology, 30*(1), 1–11.

Geddes, H. (2006). *Attachment in the Classroom: The Links Between Children's Early Experience, Emotional Well-Being and Performance in School.* London, UK: Worth Publishing.

Greenspan, S.I. (2007). *Great Kids.* Philadelphia, PA: Da Capo Press.

Hamre, B.K. & Pianta, R.C. (2007). "Learning Opportunities in Preschool and Early Elementary Classrooms." In R.C. Pianta, M.J. Cox & K.L. Snow (eds) *School Readiness and the Transition to Kindergarten in the Era of Accountability* (pp.49–83). Baltimore, MD: Paul H. Brookes Publishing Co.

Jones, D.E., Greenberg, M. & Crowley, M. (2016). "How children's social behaviors related to success in adulthood." *The WERA Educational Journal, 8*(2), 27–33.

Kertes, D.A., Kamin, H.S., Hughes, D.A., Rodney, N.C., Bhatt, S. & Mulligan, C.J. (2016). "Prenatal maternal stress predicts methylation of genes regulating the hypothalamic-pituitary-adrenocortical system in mothers and newborns in the Democratic Republic of Congo." *Child Development, 87*(10), 61–72.

Lieberman, A.F., Chu, A., Van Horn, P. & Harris, W.W. (2011). "Trauma in early childhood: Empirical evidence and clinical implications." *Development and Psychopathology, 23*(2), 397–410.

Lillas, C. & Turnbull, J. (2009). *Infant/Child Mental Health, Early Intervention, and Relationship-Based Therapies: A Neurorelational Framework for Interdisciplinary Practice.* New York, NY: W.W. Norton & Company.

Loman, M. & Gunnar, M.R. (2010). "Early experience and the development of stress reactivity and regulation in children." *Neuroscience & Biobehavioral Reviews, 34*(6), 867–876.

Luby, J., Belden, A., Botteron, K., Marrus, N. *et al.* (2013). "The effects of poverty on childhood brain development: The mediating effect of caregiving and stressful life events." *JAMA Pediatrics, 167*(12), 1135–1142.

Mashburn, A.J., Pianta, R.C., Hamre, B.K., Downer, J.T. *et al.* (2008). "Measures of classroom quality in prekindergarten and children's development of academic, language, and social skills." *Child Development, 79*(3), 732–749.

Masten, A. (2013). "Global perspectives on resilience in children and youth." *Society for Research in Child Development, 85*(1), 6–20.

Masten, A., Herbers, J., Cutuli, J. & Lafavor, T. (2008). "Promoting competence and resilience in the school context." *Professional School Counseling, 12*(2), 76–84.

McClelland, M.M. & Tominey, S.L. (2014). *The Development of Self-Regulation and Executive Function in Young Children.* Washington, DC: Zero to Three.

Murray, D.W., Rosanbalm, K., Chrisopoulos, C. & Hamoudi, A. (2015). *Self-Regulation and Toxic Stress: Foundations for Understanding Self-Regulation from an Applied Developmental Perspective.* OPRE Report #3015-21. Washington, DC: Office of Planning, Research and Evaluation, Administration for Children and Families, U.S. Department of Health and Human Services.

National Institute of Child Health and Human Development Early Child Care Research Network. (2002). "The relation of global first grade classroom environment to structural classroom features, teacher, and student behaviors." *The Elementary School Journal, 102*(5), 367–387.

National Institute of Child Health and Human Development Early Child Care Research Network. (2003). "Social functioning in first grade: Prediction from home, child care and concurrent school experience." *Child Development, 74,* 1639–1662.

National Scientific Council on the Developing Child. (2015). *Supportive Relationships and Active Skill-Building Strengthen the Foundations of Resilience: Working Paper 13.* Retrieved from www.developingchild.harvard.edu.

Oh, D.L., Jerman, P., Silverio Marques, S., Koita, K., Boparai, S.K.P., Burke-Harris, N. & Bucci, M. (2018). "Systematic review of pediatric health outcomes associated with childhood adversity." *BMC Pediatrics, 18*(83), 1–19.

Raby, K.L., Roisman, G.I., Fraley, R.C. & Simpson, J.A. (2015). "The enduring predictive significance of early maternal sensitivity: Social and academic competence through age 32 years." *Child Development, 86*(3), 695–708.

Raver, C.C. (2004). "Placing emotional self-regulation in sociocultural and socioeconomic contexts." *Child Development, 75*(2), 346–353.

Schore, A.N. (2000). "Attachment and the regulation of the right brain." *Attachment & Human Development, 2,* 23–47.

Schore, J.R. & Schore, A.N. (2008). "Modern attachment theory: The central role of affect regulation in development and treatment." *Clinical Social Work Journal, 36*(1), 9–20.

Shonkoff, J.P., Boyce, W.T. & McEwen, B.S. (2009). "Neuroscience, molecular biology, and the childhood roots of health disparities: Building a new framework for health promotion and disease prevention." *Journal of the American Medical Association, 301*(21), 2252–2259.

Silver, R.B., Measelle, J., Essex, M. & Armstrong, J.M. (2005). "Trajectories of externalizing behavior problems in the classroom: Contributions of child characteristics, family characteristics and the teacher-child relationship during the school transition." *Journal of School Psychology, 43,* 39–60.

Tucker, C., Schieffer, K., Wills, T.J., Hull, C. & Murphy, Q. (2017). "Enhancing social-emotional skills in at-risk preschool students through Theraplay based groups: The Sunshine Circle Model." *International Journal of Play Therapy, 26*(4), 185–195.

Chapter 6

Home-Based Theraplay

Annie Kiermaier

Introduction

There are many variables to consider both from the family and the practitioner's point of view when planning the most effective ways to engage a family in Theraplay. One important variable is the location. This chapter will look at home-based Theraplay intervention as an option for many families. Home-based counseling is one of the fastest-growing segments of mental health services in the US (Bowen & Caron, 2016). Home-based work has been used effectively for over a hundred years with a wide range of families with issues ranging from early intervention to working with adolescents and their families, to treating mental health issues such as depression, reducing psychiatric inpatient hospitalizations, and addressing the mental health aspects of health such as diabetes (Allen & Tracy, 2008; Carcone *et al.*, 2015; Sukhato *et al.*, 2017; Thompson *et al.*, 2009; Waisbrod, Buchbinder & Possick, 2012). The family's home can be a comfortable, familiar and convenient environment for the family. But the home can also be "complicated."

Key points

1. Home-based Theraplay can be the best location for many families, including caregivers with mental health issues (such as anxiety, depression) who are too overwhelmed to go to an office (Price, Gray & Thacker, 2014), or children who feel safer and more comfortable at home. Home-based work is especially effective

with multi-problem families (Bachler *et al.*, 2016) whose problems can adversely impact family relationships, socio-economic status and a large variety of conditions of deprivation. And home-based work can help families overcome logistical barriers to treatment such as lack of transportation, long distances to get to office-based programs, and inadequate finances to afford basic transportation (Foss, Generali & Kress, 2011; Thompson *et al.*, 2009).

2. Home-based Theraplay provides unique opportunities for the practitioner not available in an office. The practitioner is able to both objectively observe the physical and relational environment and to join with the family system in their home during sessions (Bowen & Caron, 2016; Boyd-Franklyn & Bry, 2000). This can provide opportunities for consultation and intervention that would never be possible in an office. It is an honor for the practitioner to be invited into their home and share their family, their culture and perhaps a cup of tea. Home-based work helps ensure continuity of care, accesses difficult-to-reach families, minimizes barriers, facilitates generalization of new skills and minimizes the power imbalance between family and practitioner.

3. Home-based Theraplay requires extra structure and an acceptance that daily life at home is messy and sometimes chaotic. Yes, the family dog will want to play, the TV is on and the neighbors will walk in unexpectedly. Home-based Theraplay requires careful planning and portable equipment.

4. Home-based Theraplay is "real life" and so can be a great framework for helping families integrate Theraplay into their homes.

5. The effectiveness of home-based Theraplay can actually reduce the number of sessions required and increase family participation (reduced drop-out rates) and so may actually be cost and service effective even though driving to families' homes is a consideration. And home-based Theraplay makes Theraplay accessible to families for whom office-based work would be too high a hurdle or completely impossible.

Home can be the best location for Theraplay treatment

Most people feel safe and comfortable in their own homes. Parents who struggle with mental health issues, shame-based behaviors and/or a poor internal working model may feel intimidated by walking into an office where they fear being judged and criticized. Low income and socio-economic status are correlated with depression, anxiety and generalized stress; people living in poverty access mental health services at lower rates and are more likely to prematurely discontinue treatment, in part related to heightened feelings of vulnerability and experiences of discrimination and stigma (Foss-Kelly, Generali & Kress, 2017; Price *et al.*, 2014). Home-based work allows the practitioner to reach out to vulnerable families who do not respond to traditional office-based interventions (Waisbrod *et al.*, 2012). It gives the message to the caregiver, "I am willing to come to you. I respect you. I can work with you at home where you feel most comfortable." I have worked with many caregivers who are isolated and home-bound and others whose daily schedules make office visits very difficult or impossible. For example:

- A young mother with severe depression and obesity who struggled to get herself out of bed and her child to school each day.

- Two unemployed parents with three children under the age of four with no car, no access to public transportation and no money.

- A single father with attention deficit hyperactivity disorder (ADHD) raising two young children, who could not organize himself to get to appointments at the community mental health center.

- Two professional parents with demanding jobs and two school-aged children for whom travel to my office for daytime sessions would have been one hurdle too many. The solution was early evening Family Theraplay sessions in their home followed by parent consultation.

Home-based Theraplay may also be the best location for children. Like their caregivers, they may feel most safe and comfortable at home. For most children, caregivers and home represent a child's "secure base" from which they can explore the world. Home is familiar and predictable. The child does not have to navigate the scary newness of an office with strange people and strange rooms and objects. Children who have benefited from home-based Theraplay include:

- A four-year-old girl with selective mutism living with a large extended family. Treatment was mostly with the girl and her mother, but included other family members using Group Theraplay-type family sessions.

- Two young children living with their grandmother after the death of their drug-addicted mother. The children had faced many traumas and transitions. Theraplay treatment was focused on strengthening the grandmother as their "secure base," including doing Theraplay activities in the home with their own blankets and toys.

- A nine-year-old boy struggling with anxiety and self-regulation living with his grandmother, sister and two cousins. Dyadic Theraplay with his autistic and severely anxious father (who did not live with him) helped them engage in fun, playful interactions for the first time. Dyadic Theraplay with his grandmother helped the boy co-regulate his emotional responses with her. And later, Family/Group Theraplay helped him learn how to co-regulate during family interactions in the home environment. (Home-based Theraplay allowed for dyadic Theraplay in the boy's bedroom while the young adolescent grandchild cared for the two younger grandchildren during sessions, making childcare scheduling and logistics possible.)

Deciding on home versus office-based Theraplay

Assuming you and your organization can offer families the choice between home and office-based Theraplay, here are some considerations and approaches:

- When the caregiver initially calls for help, explain that you begin with an intake interview to gather information, to get to know each other and to get written consent. Ask the caregiver if they would like the intake session to be at home or in the office. I sometimes lightheartedly say, "Remember, I'm coming to meet you, not to do a house inspection. I promise I have no white gloves!" Make clear that the intake session should, of course, be just with the caregiver, not with the child; the caregiver will need to make arrangements for the child to not be at home during the intake interview.

- During the intake interview, describe home-based versus office-based Theraplay practice and ask the caregiver where they would be most comfortable. "I can come to your home once a week and we can play together with your child on the living room floor. I'll bring a bag with some things for us to play with and a small cushion or bean-bag chair. We may also use a soft blanket that you have at home. We'll try to reduce distractions and make sure that our Theraplay time is just for you and your child: turn off the TV and the phones, put the dog outside and so on. If you choose to come to my office, I'll meet you in the waiting room and bring both of you to my office, doing a Theraplay activity, where I'll have comfy cushions for you and your child to sit on and a container of Theraplay materials. Either way, I'll be in charge of the session. All you have to do is follow my lead. We'll have time to discuss what happened and explain the Theraplay later. At home, your child might go outside and play or watch TV for a bit while we have a follow-up talk. In the office, your child might play in the waiting room or watch a movie while we talk. If that's not possible, we'll arrange another time to talk."

- An important part of the intake interview is explaining the Theraplay treatment model, including the initial sequence of sessions, and for the parent to agree to engage in the treatment. Explain that the next session will be a MIM assessment followed by a caregiver feedback session and a practice session before beginning Theraplay with the caregiver and child. Describe the importance of videoing the MIM as a way for the caregiver to see their interactions with their child from a new perspective, to give feedback to the caregiver, and to talk about treatment goals. At the family's home, you and the caregiver will look around for the best place to set up the MIM.

- Do you and your organization have the ability to move between home-based and office-based Theraplay to best meet the family's needs? Many families thrive with home-based Theraplay. But some find that the structure and lack of distractions in an office work better for them. Some parts of the work may be better suited to the home, others to the office. For instance, I worked with an eight-year-old girl to strengthen her attachment relationship with her foster parents at home, then did a sequence of sessions with her birth father during supervised visits in my office. After his parental rights were terminated because of his ongoing addiction, I resumed home-based work with her foster parents, who then adopted her.

Home-based Theraplay provides unique opportunities not available in an office

In the home, you see the family in their own environment, giving an invaluable window into daily life that is so much more real than what a caregiver might report during an intake interview in an office. Being in a family's home allows you to observe the child in their usual physical environment, the dynamics and interactions within the family system, and the influence of the surrounding culture (Allen & Tracy, 2008; Clossey *et al.*, 2018; Waisbrod *et al.*, 2012). Practitioners trained in family therapy will find observing and working in a family's home a very rich experience (Boyd-Franklin & Bry, 2000). As the Theraplay practitioner, you have the opportunity to join with the family system in the home (Stinchfield, 2004). Home-based work requires a high degree of skill, the ability to accept the family where they are, and the capacity to build a trusting relationship with them (Allen & Tracy, 2008).

For 18 years, I provided home-based mental health work to families in Maine through a non-profit early-intervention organization called Mid-Coast Children's Services. I then continued to provide some home-based work in private practice for five additional years. I cherished the unique opportunities described above as I built close and trusting relationships with families in their homes. I approach each home and family the same: with respect and deep caring for the struggles they are facing, and hopefulness that my work with them, including Theraplay, will improve their family dynamics. The simple act of coming into a family's home gives important messages: I accept you as you are; I want to understand you and the environment you live in; you honor me by letting me come into your home, your culture and your family life; we will work as a team together to make your home life better. This is especially important when we, as the practitioner, represent the mainstream or dominant culture, and the family is struggling with oppression from that dominant culture: immigrant and refugee families; families of color or mixed-race living in a predominantly white culture; low-income families who feel "less than" middle- and upper-income people; lesbian, gay or transgender families worried that they will be rejected or that they will be unsafe (Foss *et al.*, 2011; Foss-Kelly *et al.*, 2017).

Here are a few brief examples: A parent reports that the child has difficulty falling asleep at night; a home session reveals that the child's bedroom is isolated on a different floor from the parents' bedroom. A boy with significant ADHD lives in a small, cluttered house trailer with a tiny bedroom and no room to move safely; he benefits from the introduction of outdoor play time with organizing Theraplay activities. A family of four don't eat meals together because the table is piled high with mail and objects with the result that the acting-out boy runs about the house during meals. I work with the mother to clear the table and set up predictable mealtime routines where everyone sits at the table together, increasing the boy's focus and ability to stay seated. These examples illustrate that observing the home situation (bedrooms, cramped space, cluttered table) helps the practitioner understand the context of the problems with the child that would not happen in an office interview. Parents would probably not disclose that the bedrooms are far apart, that they live in a tiny trailer, or that their dining table is piled high with clutter. Actually seeing the situation helps the practitioner understand the child's problems in the context of the home environment and can either lead to problem solving with the parent (such as de-cluttering the table) or at least an understanding that the environment is having an impact on the child's behaviors, which may help the practitioner to have realistic expectations for what can be accomplished in the home.

Kate Lewer, a mental health occupational therapist and Theraplay therapist, trainer and supervisor, lives and works in Victoria, Australia. She shares the joys and struggles of doing home-based Theraplay with local Aboriginal families who are rightfully suspicious and mistrustful of "white fellas" as a result of severe oppression and genocide. Kate recalls working with "Auntie," and her two school-age nieces. Auntie chose home-based work due to her not being comfortable outside her home in a predominantly white suburb, having a history of trauma and domestic violence, and her own vision impairment that meant she could not drive a car to appointments. Auntie also cared for two extended family members. Meeting the needs of everyone in the family network was paramount to Auntie. Kate's work in the home helped her to build respect and trust with Auntie and to understand that obligation to family was a priority. In addition to Theraplay, Kate helped Auntie utilize the support of the local aboriginal community-based services. Kate needed to be flexible and patient; progress was often slow and gains seemed small (Personal communication, 2019). These opportunities for observation, consultation, building a trusting alliance and intervention would never have been possible in an office.

Home-based Theraplay can appear and feel messy and disorganized and so requires extra structure

Here are key strategies for providing structure at home:

- *Scheduling and arriving.* You schedule appointments just as you do when working in an office, but you need to get accurate directions to the family's home and plan time to arrive.

- *Appearances.* In an office, you carefully decorate and arrange the office for comfort and to create a professional atmosphere. Going to clients' homes, you need to think about the appearance of your car as well as your own appearance. Your car, believe it or not, is part of your intervention. The family and their neighbors will see you drive up and leave each week. What messages are you giving with your brand new expensive SUV or your rusty 15-year-old car? The three-year-old brother of a disabled infant threw a stone at my windshield and broke it. Handling that with the mother became part of the work. In Theraplay, we dress casually and comfortably to play with the family on the floor. Families' homes can be quite variable and unpredictable in terms of dirt and germs, so I always wear simple, comfortable, washable clothing.

- *Boundaries with neighbors.* I can guarantee confidentiality with home-based Theraplay, but not always anonymity. Neighbors may see you drive up to your client's home and want to know what's going on. You may need to talk with parents early on to anticipate how they wish to handle neighbors' questions and to ask that neighbors not interrupt Theraplay time.

- *MIM.* During the intake interview, walk about the house with the parent to find the most appropriate place to do the MIM, including where to set up your video camera. Ideally, we want to not be in the room during the MIM to reduce our possible influence on the parent-child interactions. However, in the home you have a number of things to consider. Is there a comfortable and socially appropriate place for you to wait outside the room where the MIM will happen? You may need to set clear boundaries with the parent and describe this carefully: "It looks as if you and Bobby will be most comfortable sitting at the kitchen table for the MIM. I will set up the camera and then wait in the living room until you are finished. Okay?" If being out of the room where the MIM will be happening seems socially awkward, tell the parent that you will sit quietly in the room but will try to be as unobtrusive as possible. Keep in mind how being at home might influence the "Leave the room" activity for both the parent and the child and take that into consideration when doing your MIM analysis.

- *Equipment.* What equipment do you need to do home-based Theraplay?

  - A large, sturdy bag with handles that can be closed, such as with a zipper. Keep a standard set of Theraplay resources in the bag as well as any extras that might come in handy, including hand sanitizer or wipes.

  - A small bean-bag chair with a washable surface *or* a small cushion with a removable and washable cover (dog beds are great!) for the child to sit on. You can improvise with the family's pillows and cushions; however, bringing a bean bag or cushion for the child helps to define the time and place for the Theraplay session as separate from the family's own objects.

  - A large, flat sheet (known as a "play sheet") that you can use to define the play space and have a clean surface to play on. Wash the sheet between sessions to avoid sharing dirt, germs, fleas and lice between families!

  - Do *not* bring a blanket unless you are prepared to wash it between every home session. Instead, I ask the family to provide one of their own favorite blankets.

- *Arriving and entrance activity.* Home-based Theraplay is different from office-based Theraplay because you are the one entering, not the family. From the moment you drive up to the family's home, you are defining, by your movements, your words and your equipment, that the Theraplay session is about to start. You are setting the tone and the boundaries for the session from the moment you arrive, but you also need to balance that with an understanding that you are entering their "castle" where the parent is "in charge." You carry your resource bag, cushion and play sheet up to the door and knock. After you are greeted, you have some choices:

  - Enter the home and invite the child to carry your bag and to help you set up the play space, spread the play sheet and place the resource bag and child's cushion. Put them in the same place every week.

  - Greet the parent and child and ask them to wait in another room while you prepare the designated play room (most often the living room). You might help build excitement and anticipation by calling out to them, "I'm almost ready. I'll come get you when you count slowly to 10!" Then do a traditional entrance activity with the parent and child from the room where they've been waiting into the play room.

- *Set physical, relational and time boundaries for the Theraplay session.* Because you are entering a family's home, the way your relationship with them is defined and how the space is used is totally different from office-based Theraplay. It is easy for families to think because you are coming to their home that you are their "friend." You have hopefully laid the groundwork for your professional relationship with the caregivers during the intake interview and MIM feedback session, defining your work together as using Theraplay to meet specifically defined treatment goals. You are, of course, striving to have a warm, caring, trusting relationship with the family, but you may need to remind them of your professional role and purpose for doing home-based Theraplay more than once. Some tips:

  - Set boundaries for the environment by telling the family to turn off the TV, put pets outside or in another room, turn off mobile devices, and ask family and neighbors not to visit during

Theraplay sessions. Some families have their TV on nearly all day long, so requesting to turn it off may be a significant piece of work you do with the family. You can explain: "Our Theraplay time on Tuesdays is our time to focus completely on your child without any distractions or interference." Modeling no TV during sessions may help the family to decrease TV time and create more opportunities for interactive family play during their day. I worked with a boy whose family had the TV on all day. He turned out to have severe auditory hypersensitivity. Once we understood his hypersensitivity to sound, the parents agreed to keep the TV off except for one hour a day. That intervention, along with Theraplay sessions, helped to significantly reduce the boy's angry and aggressive behaviors.

– Define play location and time: "We are going to be playing in this space where I have laid the play sheet." Place the sheet on the floor near a wall or sofa, place the child's cushion along the wall or sofa and invite the child to sit on the cushion. You may choose to close the door of the room where you are playing to prevent the child from running about the entire home. Homes are full of distractions. You may need to find an appropriate play space that is away from toys, or consider quickly covering toy areas or shelves with a sheet. You may consider asking the caregiver which areas of the home they give permission to play in. Hide and seek can be great fun in family's homes, but first carefully define which rooms to use. "Mom, can we play hide and seek in the kitchen, living room, bathroom and Bobby's bedroom today?" One great advantage of home-based Theraplay is the ability to do Theraplay outdoors. "Red light/ Green light" and "Mother may I" are fantastic to play outside the home if the child is able to respond to adult-led structure. If a caregiver is struggling with providing age-appropriate structure for their child, home-based Theraplay sessions may be initially quite challenging. But the strengthening of parent-led structure can be lasting. Because this is in the family's home, you will need to define the beginning and the end of the session. It may help to do the same initial and ending activity each week.

You might begin with a special greeting song while you begin the Check-In, sitting closely in front of the child ("Shakira's here today, Shakira's here today, let's clap our hands and shout Hooray! Shakira's here today!"). You might end by putting the child's shoes back on and saying, "Our special Theraplay time is all done today! That was fun!"

– "The adult is in charge." This is, of course, one of the key Theraplay principles, but it is especially important when doing home-based Theraplay. The adult-led Theraplay session may be very different from the way the parent and child interact during the rest of their week at home. You may need to define the structure and adult-led nature of Theraplay to the parent and child: "We have our special Theraplay time every week in your bedroom. When we do Theraplay together I will lead play activities that I think will be fun and helpful for both of you. All you both have to do is relax and have fun! It may be different from the rest of your week together, but I think it's going to be a good time." Like office-based Theraplay, you can tell the caregiver that sessions will begin with the practitioner being in charge, with a gradual shift to the caregiver guiding the Theraplay activities as their understanding of Theraplay and their confidence grow. Because the Theraplay is in the family's home, you may sometimes need to defer to caregiver authority at home and focus on a caregiver-practitioner team approach. For example, if a child leaves the session, you may ask the caregiver, "How shall we handle this?"

– Relational boundaries. You have been honored to be welcomed into a family's home and family life. Do you accept a cup of coffee or a home-made cookie? (Answer: it depends on the meaning of the cup of coffee or the cookie to each individual family.) Again, families can read your warmth and playfulness as you being their friend. Or they may be testing to see if you genuinely accept them and their culture, especially if their culture is oppressed and you represent the dominant culture, such as families of color, immigrant families, families dealing with poverty, or LGBT families. They may ask you personal questions. They may give you gifts at Christmas or at the end of treatment. An occasional hand-drawn picture or a small token can be accepted graciously ("Thank you. I'll put that on my desk at my office"). But setting clear boundaries may be difficult at times: "I'm sorry, but I can't give you a ride to the grocery store after our session. It's really not part of our work and my agency doesn't allow employees to transport people in their cars." You may need to define the working relationship you have: "I'm so glad that you enjoy our Theraplay time together each week and that you see me as a friendly person who cares about you. Some things we do together may feel like what friends do. But there's a difference: even though our time is warm and friendly, I am always working to help your family life be better. I am only here for a short time. Your family is with you forever." Like office-based Theraplay, you may need to anticipate with families how you will greet each other when you meet at the grocery store or somewhere else in town, especially if you live and work in a small community.

- *Caregiver consultation time.* One great advantage of home-based Theraplay is that it can be easier to have time to debrief and consult with the caregiver than it is in the office. After a 30+ minute Theraplay session, the child can be invited to go play outside or in their bedroom, to play with siblings or neighbors, or to watch a favorite TV program or movie while you sit in another room and talk with the caregiver. The child may occasionally return to the kitchen to see what Mom and you are doing, but often returns to play or TV because that grownup talk is boring. This works well for many children, but can be difficult if the child has significant self-regulation problems such as ADHD or if the child is hypervigilant or has insecure, anxious attachment. If so, you may need to follow up with a phone call or an additional appointment to consult with the caregiver.

- *Safety.* Most home-based Theraplay can feel quite adventurous and fun. But occasionally there can be threats and dangers to the practitioner (Allen & Tracy, 2008). Key tips:

  - Carefully assess the safety of the home and the neighborhood.

- Try to predict possible safety issues and prevent them from happening ahead of time.

- As mentioned above, set clear physical, time and relational boundaries. Follow your organization's procedures on home visits. Keep your phone with you.

- If a difficulty arises, your safety is the priority. If necessary, leave the situation.

- If necessary, give someone in your organization your schedule, including times and addresses of your home visits. Make it clear if you are headed to a possible unsafe situation. Tell your organization that if you do not call in after the home visit that they are to try to call you and then to call the police. In all my years of home-based work, I have arranged this with my organization only a handful of times, but never felt unsafe enough to initiate calling the police.

I worked with young parents of two toddlers. The father had a history of assaulting a public health nurse who came to their home. I always kept myself between the father and the door to their apartment so that I could leave quickly if his temper escalated. Fortunately, it never did.

As I've said, the home-based practitioner needs to understand that "real" family life is complex. Home-based Theraplay will often be a bit messy and less structured than in an office setting, but the advantage of immediately integrating Theraplay into the home usually outweighs the "messy" disadvantages. Home-based Theraplay requires the practitioner to be attuned, adaptable, flexible and tolerant of "real life." These are exactly the characteristics we hope for the families we work with.

Home-based Theraplay can be the perfect way to help families integrate Theraplay into their environment, relationships, culture and home routines

- *Environment.* During Theraplay sessions, use the resources in the home environment. Rock the child in a favorite blanket. Stack the sofa cushions high for a structured jumping challenge. Use a favorite toy for a bean-bag drop. Blow cotton balls with straws across the kitchen table. This way, when it is time to encourage caregivers to do Theraplay themselves, the materials at home will already be a familiar part of the suggested activities. During caregiver consultation time, the practitioner and parent can look about the home to brainstorm ways to integrate Theraplay.

- *Relationships.* Activities done during home-based Theraplay can naturally emerge during interactions between family members. A parent may wink at a child who then winks back or responds with a silly face. A child may ask a caregiver to sing "Twinkle, twinkle." A caregiver may do a four-part handshake with his child before leaving for work in the morning. Many families live in cultures that encourage large extended families to care for and support each other. Grandparents, aunts/uncles and cousins may share a household or live nearby. Home-based Theraplay gives you the opportunity to observe and understand the family system and how it can support or perhaps hinder your work to strengthen the family relationships.

- *Culture.* Understanding, accepting and respecting the family's culture is an essential part of home-based Theraplay, most especially if the family's culture is different than the dominant culture. If the family's culture is different from your own, you will need to do "homework" to anticipate how to integrate Theraplay into the family. For example, working with immigrant families who speak a different language and who have different customs and ways of relating can be challenging but also very rewarding. Working with cultures or religious groups that have strict rules about contact between genders requires some adaptations. Asking the family to teach you their traditional songs and simple games that can be incorporated into Theraplay can help the family understand that Theraplay can work within their culture and can help you build trust and respect for the family's culture.

- *Home routines.* Working in the home, it's easier to imagine the flow of routines throughout the day and then support the family to integrate Theraplay into their daily routines. Perhaps they'll do a family hand stack around the kitchen table before dinner. Or do a weather report adaptation for a child at bedtime. The practitioner may also recommend more structured Theraplay sessions and work with the caregiver to identify the best time and place in the home for those special play times. *Parenting with Theraplay* by Vivien Norris and Helen Rodwell (2017) is an excellent resource for caregivers, describing Theraplay in caregiver-friendly language and providing many ideas for integrating Theraplay into their family lives.

Home-based Theraplay may actually be cost and service effective even though driving to families' homes is a consideration

You and your organization will need to plan into your work schedule the time it takes to drive to families' homes as well as the expense of driving your car or taking public transportation. But remember to balance the time and cost with the accessibility, effectiveness and lower drop-out rates of home-based Theraplay for many families, as evidenced by the case presented below.

 ## CASE ILLUSTRATION
BACKGROUND

Theo was born to an alcohol- and drug-dependent single mother who struggled to care for him. His maternal grandparents, Bob and Sue, were active participants in his care when he was an infant. When he was nine months old, Child Protection Services placed Theo in his grandparents' care because of his mother's ongoing addiction and dangerous behaviors. Bob and Sue later received permanency guardianship. Both grandparents worked full time, each driving 30–45 minutes in different directions to work each day. Four-year-old Theo was developmentally delayed and extremely hyperactive and impulsive. His grandparents were exhausted and frustrated and often resorted to yelling at Theo to "STOP!" which had little effect. He attended childcare near Bob's work, so Bob transported him each day.

THERAPLAY PROCESS AND PROGRESSION

Home-based Theraplay sessions were scheduled for 5:30pm weekly, just as Sue arrived home from work. She and I had 20–30 minutes to review last week's Theraplay session and consult on managing Theo's behaviors. Then Theo would arrive with his grandfather, bounding into the home and ready for Theraplay. Co-regulation was, of course, the primary goal. Theo would jump into my bean-bag chair that was propped against the sofa. Sue and I would sit on the floor facing him and together take off his shoes. Structured Theraplay sessions were short (20–25 minutes) and intense, always starting with a lively Check-In with lots of proprioceptive input (squeezing hands, high-fives, etc.), building to a single peak of structured activity such as Red light/Green light, then tapering down the intensity, ending with a feeding activity that involved lots of active, loud crunching and sipping vigorously from a sport bottle. Lastly, we always ended with rocking Theo in the blanket while singing *Twinkle, Twinkle Little Star*, his favorite part of the sessions. We ended by telling him what was happening next at home, which was usually dinner.

Some sessions involved just Sue while Bob prepared dinner. Other times, dinner was ready in the crock-pot or quickly microwaved and Bob either observed or joined in the play. Bob especially enjoyed the active play. Theo's toys were piled up in a corner of the living room. Sometimes he would reach for a large toy truck. I would make it into a structured activity, telling him to roll it to Bob on the count of "1, 2, 3, GO!" and Bob would roll it back to Theo and me, then we would repeat. Theo became better able to follow adult-led directions and to regulate his activity level. Bob and Sue learned how to provide structured play that helped co-regulate Theo. They learned to build that lively and structured approach into their daily interactions with Theo, including how to take turns with him so they didn't get so exhausted. In the warmer months when there was still daylight in the early evening, Theo, Bob and I would play outside in the yard, often starting with unstructured gross motor play, then building in more structure and gradually reducing the activity level as we returned inside.

OUTCOME

After nine months of weekly sessions, Theo remained a lively, active boy but his grandparents were able to keep him within a healthy "window of tolerance" much more of the time than when we first met. Life was much more manageable and their relationships were warm and fun.

Conclusion

Theo and his grandparents responded well to home-based Theraplay. It met their busy work and travel needs; coming to an office would have had to have been a 7pm session and required an extra hour of travel for them on busy work days, making treatment virtually impossible for them and much more difficult for me as the practitioner (Foss *et al.*, 2011). Theo's grandparents were able to learn the concept of co-regulation and the need for structure and build these into their physical environment and daily routines. Like many families, home-based Theraplay was accessible and adaptable for Theo's family.

Questions for reflection and continued learning

1. How will your intake protocol determine if home-based Theraplay might be best for a family? You might consider asking yourself, "Why *not* do home-based Theraplay?"

2. What are some important observations and interventions you might be able to do at home that could never happen in your office? How will you structure your home-based Theraplay sessions?

3. How can you help families to integrate Theraplay into their home environment and routines?

References

Allen, S.F. & Tracy, E.M. (2008). "Developing student knowledge and skills for home-based social work practice." *Journal of Social Work Education, 44*(1), 125–143.

Bachler, E., Frühmann, A., Bachler, H., Aas, B., Strunk, G. & Nickel, M. (2016). "Differential effects of the working alliance in family therapeutic home-based treatment of multi-problem families." *Journal of Family Therapy, 38*, 120–148.

Bowen, J. & Caron, S.L. (2016). "A qualitative analysis of home-based counselors' experiences in a rural setting." *Journal of Counseling & Development, 94*, 129–140.

Boyd-Franklin, N. & Bry, B.H. (2000). *Reaching Out in Family Therapy: Home-Based, School, and Community Interventions*. New York, NY: Guilford Press.

Carcone, A.I., Ellis, D.A., Chen, X., Naar, S., Cunningham, P.B. & Moltz, K. (2015). "Multisystemic therapy improves the patient-provider relationship in families of adolescents with poorly controlled insulin dependent diabetes." *Journal of Clinical Psychology in Medical Settings, 22*, 169–178.

Clossey, L., Simms, S., Hu, C., Hartzell, J., Duah, P. & Daniels, L. (2018). "A pilot evaluation of the rapid response program: A home-based family therapy." *Community Mental Health Journal, 54*, 302–311.

Foss, L.L., Generali, M.M. & Kress, V.E. (2011). "Counseling people living in poverty: The CARE Model." *Journal of Humanistic Counseling, 50*, 161–171.

Foss-Kelly, L.L., Generali, M.M. & Kress, V.E. (2017). "Counseling strategies for empowering people living in poverty: The I-CARE Model." *Journal of Multicultural Counseling and Development, 45*, 201–213.

Norris, V. & Rodwell, H. (2017). *Parenting with Theraplay*. London, UK: Jessica Kingsley Publishers.

Price, S.H., Gray, L.A. & Thacker, L.R. (2014). "Enhanced engagement: An intervention pilot for mental health promotion among low-income women in a community home visiting program." *Best Practices in Mental Health, 11*(1), 69–82.

Stinchfield, T.A. (2004). "Clinical competencies specific to family-based therapy." *Counselor Education & Supervision, 43*, 286–300.

Sukhato, K., Lotrakul, M., Dellow, A., Ittasakul, P., Thakkinstian, A. & Anothaisintawee, T. (2017). "Efficacy of home-based non-pharmacological interventions for treating depression: A systematic review and network meta-analysis of randomized controlled trials." *British Medical Journal Open, 7*, 1–15.

Thompson, S.J., Bender, K., Windsor, L.C. & Flynn, P.M. (2009). "Keeping families engaged: The effects of home-based family therapy enhanced with experiential activities." *Social Work Research, 33*(2), 121–126.

Waisbrod, N., Buchbinder, E. & Possick, C. (2012). "In-home intervention with families in distress: Changing places to promote change." *Social Work, 57*(2), 121–132.

Chapter 7

Theraplay Adaptations for Anxiety Disorders

Danielle H. Maxonight

Introduction

This chapter explores the benefits of Theraplay for anxious children and their caregivers. Although the *Diagnostic and Statistical Manual of Mental Disorders* (*DSM-5*) recognizes important distinctions among anxiety disorders, here I will reference "anxiety disorders" more broadly. Many overlaps exist; indeed, within treatment-seeking populations, up to 75 percent of children with one anxiety disorder will meet criteria for two or more (Costello *et al.*, 2003). The therapeutic needs of this population will be examined within existing literature, and Theraplay adaptations will be illustrated. Lastly, common presenting concerns and therapeutic approaches will be contextualized in a case study.

Key points

1. A secure, authoritative caregiver-child relationship and robust caregiver coaching within treatment will lead to the best outcomes for children with anxiety. As such, Theraplay is an ideal intervention.

2. Anxiety disorders are often intergenerational. Effective therapy must tend to the needs of both children and caregivers.

3. Central themes of treatment are predictability and role definition.

4. We must adapt protocol to meet a dyad's unique needs. In the case

of a child's separation anxiety, we include their caregiver in all play sessions. For highly anxious caregivers, we increase our availability and approach as needed.

Theraplay with anxious children: theoretical underpinnings
Caregiver-child relationship

Theraplay operates within the notion that the caregiver-child relationship drives change; but how does a caregiver's behavior, parenting or attachment style impact their child's anxiety disorder? Is a healthy relationship curative? And how much influence do caregivers really have?

Parenting style

Researchers agree that the parenting approach correlative with anxiety in children involves three main areas of concern: overprotection, intrusiveness and negativity (McLeod, Wood & Weisz, 2007). As attachment-based practitioners, we also recognize that parent and child emotional states and behaviors reverberate off of one another, creating patterned interactions that take on a life of their own. This makes it difficult to ascertain which came first, the child anxiety or the parenting behavior. Some theorize that a child's naturally inhibited temperament may elicit more overprotection from parents, thereby exacerbating a child's anxiety in a cycle that intensifies the responses of both dyad members over time (Hudson & Rapee, 2004; Rubin, Coplan & Bowker, 2009). Theraplay seeks to break this cycle. We focus on restructuring relational patterns that no longer serve the caregiver-child dyad.

Parents can significantly temper the impact of childhood anxiety, if not completely resolve it, through particular types of interactions with their children. Diana Baumrind delineated four parenting styles—indulgent, authoritarian, authoritative and uninvolved—each with varying levels of parental demandingness (*structure*) and responsiveness (*nurture*). An authoritative parent has a strong balance of both: she "enforces her own perspective as an adult, but recognizes the child's individual interests and special ways… [She] does not base her decisions on group consensus or the individual child's desires" but on the child's needs, and she responds to feelings in a warm, connected way (Baumrind, 1967, pp.890–891). This structure/nurture balance is a desired outcome of all Theraplay interventions, and, in fact, research on the authoritative style is one of the bases for the adult-guided nature of the model (Booth & Lindaman, 2010). An authoritative parenting style has been found to significantly moderate childhood anxiety, leading to fewer internalizing behavior problems (Paulussen-Hoogeboom *et al.*, 2008; Williams *et al.*, 2009), increased psychological flexibility (Williams, Ciarrochi & Heaven, 2012), less maladaptive perfectionism (Hibbard & Walton, 2014), more adaptive social behavior (Rinaldia & Howe, 2012) and less social inhibition (Rubin, Burgess & Hastings, 2002), when compared with other parenting styles. This healthy, warm-but-firm parenting approach is modeled, scaffolded and reinforced throughout the Theraplay intervention.

Attachment style

Furthermore, given the relationship between insecure attachment and anxiety, Theraplay's focus on fostering security is a worthy goal. Indeed, a number of researchers propose that insecure attachment is the primary mediating factor between parenting style and anxiety disorders in later life (Schimmenti & Bifulco, 2013). Meta-analysis of 46 studies—over more than three decades of research—found that insecurity is moderately related to anxiety, with ambivalent attachment showing the strongest correlation (Colonnesi *et al.*, 2011). Insecure attachment patterning has been correlated with childhood anxiety, even independent of maternal anxiety. Prenatal maternal anxiety is an established contributor to child emotional problems (Van den Bergh *et al.*, 2005); however, in a study of over one hundred at-risk three- to four-year-olds, an insecure mother-child attachment, as measured by the Strange Situation Protocol, was independently associated with child anxiety disorders, even when controlling for maternal anxiety (Shamir-Essakow, Ungerer & Rapee, 2005). This finding offers hope for attachment-based interventions such as Theraplay in that the children's anxiety was not predetermined by the mother's anxiety process on its own, but rather, the mother-child attachment.

Parentification

Although "childhood anxiety" may conjure the image of a withdrawn, inhibited child, we recognize that anxiety can present relationally in a number of other ways, including a child's defiant, controlling or caretaking behavior with a parent. Enmeshed boundaries and emotional parentification have been found to correlate with later internalizing disorders (Jacobvitz *et al.*, 2004; Katz, Petracca & Rabinowitz, 2009; Tan *et al.*, 2010). This underscores the effectiveness of intervening at the level of the dyad, building strong role definitions and emotional boundaries between parent and child. Theraplay addresses these issues robustly.

Parental involvement in treatment

Surprisingly, parental involvement in child-focused cognitive behavioral therapy (CBT) has not consistently led to better outcomes, perhaps because the type of involvement can vary so widely (Breinholst *et al.*, 2012). A study comparing various types of parental inclusion found that children had the best long-term outcomes when their parents learned specific interventions to use at home. Teaching hands-on skills and transferring control from the therapist to the parent helped maintain treatment gains and even decrease the children's anxiety more over time, relative to other forms of involvement (Manassis *et al.*, 2014). Theraplay follows a similar trajectory of parent coaching and empowerment, adding in direct practice of the new parenting responses in real time during play sessions.

Genetic factors

Although caregivers can have a significant impact on moderating their child's anxiety, it is essential to recognize that anxiety disorders have an undeniable hereditary component. Adults with anxiety are more likely to have children with anxiety, and vice versa (Rapee, Schniering & Hudson, 2009). Setting aside the environmental influences on intergenerational transmission of anxiety (such as parenting or attachment style), researchers estimate that between 30 and 40 percent of the variance in anxiety symptoms and diagnoses are mediated by genetics (Gregory & Eley, 2007). Educating caregivers about hereditary risk factors can relieve them of feeling too responsible for their child's struggles. This is important information to integrate into treatment planning and parent psychoeducation.

Existing research

A small but promising body of research builds support for Theraplay's effectiveness with childhood anxiety disorders. In a 2011 study of 167 practitioner-child dyads, Theraplay reduced social withdrawal and increased self-confidence, assertiveness and expressive and receptive communication in children with social anxiety (Wettig, Coleman & Geider, 2011). Both Group Theraplay and Sunshine Circles, a group therapy adaptation of Theraplay for preschoolers, also show great potential. The Sunshine Circles intervention improved children's prosocial behavior and reduced anxiety (Tucker *et al.*, 2017), and eight weeks of Group Theraplay resulted in fewer internalizing symptoms in a high-risk sample of second, third and fourth graders, when compared with a waitlist control group (Siu, 2009).

Theraplay with anxious children: treatment themes and adaptations

Given the skill required to co-regulate arousal and manage resistance (see Chapter 1), most Theraplay practitioners will already have many tools to confidently and effectively treat anxiety disorders in children. Here I will discuss treatment themes and creative adaptations to further enhance outcomes for this population.

Increasing predictability

Anxious children have both a heightened expectation of threat (Schniering & Lyneham, 2007) and a tendency to interpret ambiguous information as threatening (Muris & Field, 2013). Because of this, we focus on structure: building emotional safety through predictable, clear and consistent sequences of activities. We establish routines to help the dyad better manage anxious states. Discovering particularly enjoyable or effective activities, we remember these comforting rituals from the first few Theraplay sessions and then repeat them as needed throughout treatment.

We use rituals to support transitions, when anxiety is high. For example, during the transition from the waiting area into the office, a practitioner might follow a familiar routine of carrying a child on piggyback to a soft pillow, exclaiming that a special constellation of freckles "is still in the same perfect spot!" and singing a welcome song. A shoe race in which the practitioner always loses dramatically to the caregiver might indicate the end of session, while the transition from office back to lobby is shored up through the use of a Lycra tunnel. The practitioner gives a high-five to the child in their office while the caregiver waits at the other side of the tunnel in the lobby, calling "1, 2, 3, crawl to me!"

We must be deliberate with even the smallest transitions while working with this population, using "first, then" statements and verbal warnings between activities: "First we'll do two more big jumps, then we'll move on to another activity. Wow, that was a huge jump! That was jump number one. Let's do our last jump now!" A child's initial hesitation at the outset of a brand-new activity may be eased by first demonstrating the activity with the caregiver. This adds a layer of emotional safety for the child as they consider venturing into the new experience.

At the beginning of treatment, the level of predictability must match the child's level of anxiety in order to unburden the child. For profoundly anxious children, this may mean multiple sessions of almost entirely replicated sequences of activities. Other children may need to see a written or picture schedule. Still others will respond best to having materials spread out on the floor, rather than hidden mysteriously in the practitioner's bag (Glibota, Lindaman & Coleman, 2018). Each child is unique; the goal in treatment planning is to create just enough certainty to build emotional safety, without placing the child in a position of authority or compromising healthy structure.

As we establish a pattern of effective co-regulation and trust, we can slowly increase the level of spontaneity, relying on the security of the new attachment patterning to gently stretch the child's nervous system. A child's ability to respond to novelty with resilience is a powerful marker of secure attachment (Schore, 2009). If a child responds to novelty with great anxiety or resistance, then "normal" rituals should be resumed temporarily. Ultimately, it is in the child's best interest to develop some level of adaptability, given that family life and the world at large are unpredictable; however, this process of developing security and resilience should never be rushed. Predictability is like a safe harbor to which practitioners and families can return again and again as needed.

Increasing role definition

As previously discussed, problems with role definition in childhood are connected to anxiety later on. Theraplay sessions offer endless opportunities to delineate, restructure and reinforce healthy child and caregiver roles. Our intent is to relieve the child of the heavy burden of taking on the adult's leadership role. This is especially important for anxious children who struggle with controlling behavior or over-responsibility. The practitioner, and later on in treatment the caregiver, must take ownership for initiating activities and determining the duration, pacing and intensity of activities in order to meet the child's needs. This involves responsiveness and attunement, as well as planning.

The practitioner might announce, "Let's keep this balloon in the air with only our knees!" After noticing the child struggling with the task and making erratic grunting noises, the practitioner repairs and amends her earlier idea: "I made this way too tricky. I know how to make this more fun! Let's use our pointer fingers and try to keep it going for three hits. 1, 2, 3, wow!" The practitioner is a calm, confident leader and responds to the child's need for mastery. A child whose needs are being met through an activity but who makes demands, changes the rules or attempts to switch roles with the adults elicits a different response. Recognizing that this child is resisting or "testing out" the new, healthy interactional pattern, the practitioner reinforces her original idea while supporting the child emotionally. In essence, we must work to meet the child's need, rather than the child's whim.

Some anxious children need firm limits around taking on inappropriate caregiving roles or "undoing" nurture by reflexively "paying back" activities to their caregiver. For example, a child who has been given a band-aid for a scrape announces, "Now I'll put a band-aid on your hand too, Mommy!" The practitioner redirects in a warm and playful, melodic tone, "In here, parents take care of kids. Kids don't take care of parents." We reinforce the special one-directional nature of caregiving in many ways, such as making sure that the caregiver stands first and helps the child to stand, the caregiver feeds the child, the caregiver puts lotion on the child's hand and so on. If the caregiver is in need of nurture, the practitioner takes on this role, rather than permitting the child to take care of their caregiver.

Adapting for separation anxiety

We never force children with fears about separation to participate in Theraplay without their caregiver. Instead, we adapt the standard protocol to involve caregivers physically—without imposing a premature leadership role on the caregiver or derailing treatment. During the caregiver demonstration session, we inform the caregiver of their initial role and encourage the caregiver to follow our lead at the beginning and middle phases of treatment. Most caregivers are happy to relinquish some responsibility and allow us to guide the play sessions. At the beginning of treatment, the caregiver will serve mostly as support for their child in terms of offering physical proximity and touch. We also demonstrate an activity with the caregiver in order to increase predictability, as a precursor to child participation. Providing much verbal direction in play sessions, the practitioner lets the caregiver know, "I want you to stand right here on this spot, and your child can stand right in front of you, holding hands. Great!" We also offer physical guidance through hand-over-hand support. For example, holding the caregiver's hands in her own, the therapist demonstrates a less ticklish quality of touch during the "weather report" activity.

Adapting for caregiver anxiety

In many ways, work with caregiver anxiety parallels work with child anxiety. Clearly defined roles and predictability are key. Given that the first few play sessions will be quite unpredictable for both caregiver and practitioner, the prolonged assessment phase serves a key function: establishing the practitioner as a nurturing and trustworthy guide for the caregiver. The level of security within the caregiver-practitioner relationship will determine much of the overall effectiveness of Theraplay treatment. Theraplay requires caregivers to venture outside their typical ways of parenting, utilizing the practitioner as a secure base from which to explore new interactional patterns and as a safe haven to return to for comfort. If the caregiver's ability to use our support in this way is compromised in any way, additional caregiver-only work can be an effective foundation before beginning the Theraplay treatment.

Anxious caregivers thrive in conditions of predictability. Practitioners coach caregivers in their own sessions to predict their child's responses (and their own responses) to the activities early and often. Developing predictions, including worst-case scenarios, is particularly essential with regard to weathering the resistance phase. For some dyads, the caregiver anxiety generated by child behaviors is preventing change. In these cases, both the child and the caregiver will present with a form of resistance. Caregivers might voice frequent doubts about therapy, fears that child behaviors will worsen indefinitely, or concerns that their child's mild, tolerable discomfort in a session is psychologically harmful. Some caregivers will undermine us in play sessions or cancel frequently. Without support, these caregivers typically end treatment during the resistance phase. It is extraordinarily important to prepare caregivers for resistance, to wonder with caregivers how they might feel and act during this phase, and to strengthen their resolve throughout this period of increased discomfort. This helps caregivers understand and contain their own elevated anxiety in order to persevere.

In some settings, two Theraplay practitioners work as a team, allowing the practitioner with the caregiver to have more opportunities to process the sessions immediately. However, the more typical situation is that one practitioner works with the dyad, and extensive processing is delayed until the caregiver-only session following three dyadic sessions. This delay will be difficult for an anxious caregiver and may even compromise their trust in us or jeopardize the entire therapeutic process. For these caregivers, we increase our availability between sessions if possible. Doing so will prevent many complex treatment issues. It is also advisable to initiate contact with a caregiver in order to provide reassurance and containment if their child displays strongly resistant behaviors or if the caregiver is observably distressed during a play session. Regardless of our chosen format for between-session contact, we must communicate within firm boundaries, in a very consistent, structured fashion that has been previously outlined with the caregiver. For instance, the practitioner might encourage email contact (compliant with the Health Insurance Portability and Accountability Act) between sessions as needed and inform the caregiver that all emails will be responded to within 48 hours, via a ten-minute phone call. If the caregiver reaches out frequently or the practitioner is unable to provide between-session contact, this may signal the need for additional caregiver-only sessions. In offering emotional co-regulation, encouragement and consistency of response will go a long way in strengthening a caregiver's inner stability and commitment to therapy. This frees up the caregiver to explore the new "Theraplay way" of responding to their child.

CASE ILLUSTRATION
BRIEF CASE BACKGROUND

Maisie was a white seven-year-old girl meeting criteria for generalized anxiety disorder and separation anxiety disorder. Although she would not meet criteria for PTSD, she suffered from specific phobias (needles, hospitals, doctors), probably resulting from medical trauma. During immunizations, Maisie would panic, scream and hide under the doctor's table for hours as her mother begged her to cooperate. She presented as eager-to-please and pseudo mature within her school setting; however, before school, Maisie was tearful, clinging and pleading with her mother to stay at home. Occasionally, she experienced panic attacks. She avoided walking through her house without her mother in eyesight.

SESSION 1: COMPREHENSIVE CLINICAL ASSESSMENT

In the first session, I met alone with the parents, Clarissa and John, to explore Maisie's needs. Maisie had been the product of a planned but high-stress pregnancy; she was born medically fragile and required several painful, invasive medical interventions in her first year. Despite much effort on her parents' part, Maisie had never successfully slept in her own bed throughout the night. Both parents had resigned themselves to co-sleeping. I described the dyadic nature of Theraplay, and we all agreed that treatment would focus on the maternal relationship. I prepared the family for the Adult Attachment Interview (AAI) in the following session. I described the importance of understanding Maisie's "half of the equation," as well as Clarissa's inner landscape, in order to best support their relationship.

SESSION 2: ADULT ATTACHMENT INTERVIEW

Clarissa recounted growing up in an unstable, narcissistic family system, suffering profound emotional neglect and childhood anxiety related to an explosive, unpredictable father. She received CBT in early adulthood, with good effect. In response to questions about her dreams for Maisie, Clarissa broke into a dewy-eyed smile: "I hope one day she is able to feel free of her anxiety. She comes by it honestly though, with me for a mom. Poor thing!"

In processing the interview together, Clarissa and I were able to draw a parallel between the trauma Clarissa experienced in her family of origin, and the way Maisie's fearful clinging activated her own anxiety in the present. This generated a great deal of self-compassion. I also shored up Clarissa's confidence by highlighting some of her parenting strengths: her willingness to seek support for Maisie, her self-reflective nature, and her own work in CBT. Challenging Clarissa's all-or-nothing belief that her parenting was the sole cause of Maisie's problems, I noted a likely hereditary component and early medical procedures as important risk factors: "a perfect storm."

SESSIONS 3–4: MIM AND FEEDBACK SESSIONS

In the next sessions, I guided Clarissa and Maisie through the MIM. I reviewed and analyzed the videotape, identifying strengths and possible areas for focus.

As Clarissa had come to treatment with shame and anxiety around her parenting abilities, I made an effort to praise her and to point out the ways she had differentiated from her family of origin. I showed her video clips that illustrated how Clarissa had truly become "a totally new kind of parent." I also provided education on the four dimensions of Theraplay and selected a weaker clip. In this segment, Clarissa attempted to put lotion on Maisie's hand, but Maisie seemed unable to be calm, first verbally directing and scolding her mother and then flipping upside down, somersaulting across the floor. I paused the tape and asked Clarissa to reflect on her own feelings and her daughter's in that moment. Clarissa said, "Maisie is really sensitive. I think the lotion freaked her out, and she was really nervous being in a new place. I was feeling embarrassed and overwhelmed too, as if maybe I'm just not cut out for parenting. I didn't really know what to do." After providing empathy for how difficult it was to experience and share those feelings, I spent some time discussing how anxiety can drive children towards more controlling behavior, and how structure can help alleviate anxiety. I said, "Even though Maisie might reject it at first, she probably needs even more structure than the average kid because she is so anxious. This can be really tricky for parents, because often the kids who need it the most resist it the hardest! So, it feels very counterintuitive and confusing sometimes. Let's try to figure it out together. I also think if we can find some types of touch that feel good to Maisie, touch will help her feel calmer." We agreed that nurture and structure should be areas for focus.

SESSION 5: PARENT DEMONSTRATION SESSION

Clarissa and John came together next for some experiential learning. I supported each parent in receiving and leading activities. Clarissa expressed personal discomfort around the close proximity and touch elements, but she imagined her daughter enjoying the attention.

I carefully prepared parents for the overall trajectory of treatment. I discussed an initial "getting to know each other" phase, the potential for Maisie to experience discomfort with the new ways of interacting, integration of the new interactional patterns, and the gradual shift from the practitioner to Clarissa as the primary leader in sessions. I reassured Clarissa that at the start of treatment she could "relax and let me take the lead. I will be responsible for structuring things and responding to behaviors." Because of Clarissa's history of anxiety, I spent extra time imagining with her the many ways in which Maisie might express resistance and ways I might respond therapeutically.

SESSIONS 6–9: THERAPLAY SESSIONS

In the first play session, I met both Clarissa and Maisie in the lobby. Little Maisie hung on to her mother's leg with a distressed look, so I encouraged the pair to lock arms and tiptoe as quietly as possible together into the therapy office. "Clarissa, you can sit right here on these pillows and Maisie can plop right in your lap facing out towards me. Yes! How snuggly! You can give her a big squeeze now!" I said. Maisie beamed and nuzzled into her mom further. Then I sang a special "hello song" to welcome the pair. Since Clarissa had expressed nervousness around touch, I asked for her permission before engaging Maisie directly: "Is it okay if I play some games with your daughter today?" I guided the dyad through bean-bag drop, placing Mom's hands beneath Maisie's so that they could participate as a team. The physical touch, steady rhythm and predictability of Clarissa's movements allowed her daughter to slowly relax her arms and go with the flow of the activity. Maisie's initial nervousness settled into more connected eye contact and less clinging throughout the first session. She sighed, giving me a sad look at the end.

In the second session, I sang the same welcome song and orchestrated the same closing ritual of blanket swing, pizza on the back, and feeding the same type of fruit snacks. Maisie seemed more comfortable as she participated in these familiar activities while near her mom but not requiring constant physical contact with her. After only two play sessions, Clarissa reported that Maisie seemed less anxious overall; in fact, she had elected to sleep in her own bed the past two nights, to the parents' great surprise. Maisie said, "When I have worry thoughts at night, I just push them away and choose a new thought." This was a CBT skill that Clarissa had been attempting to teach her daughter for several months without success.

SESSION 10: PARENT REVIEW AND FEEDBACK SESSION

In addition to discussing the ongoing sleep issue, I shared several video clips with Clarissa and John. Together we noticed the many small ways Maisie expressed her anxiety, including overly silly behavior, a shrill laugh and attempts to direct her mother. We noted that when I used more proximity, structuring touch, predictable sequences of activities and a firm-yet-warm tone of voice, Maisie seemed calmer and more cooperative.

We also explored structure experientially. I helped Clarissa first follow and then lead the Mirror activity with John. Both parents discovered that they felt more relaxed following as opposed to leading. Clarissa reflected that this concept and felt sense of structure was new and important, as her own parents had led through fear, and she did not want to replicate their abuse with Maisie.

SESSIONS 11–15: THERAPLAY SESSIONS

I continued to focus on down-regulating strategies for Maisie and on modeling healthy structure for Clarissa. By session 13, Maisie was experiencing more resistance. In sessions, she often commanded her mother, attempted to initiate or direct activities, and became very upset when words to the standard welcome song were slightly altered. To my amazement, outside the sessions, Maisie's anxiety significantly decreased. She had been able to tolerate several visits to her sick aunt, despite her extreme fear of hospitals. Maisie also slept in her own bed for stretches of three or more days during this period.

SESSION 16: PARENT REVIEW

Her parents reported that Maisie was now sleeping in her own bed consistently and had not had a panic attack in over a month. Clarissa shared that she had noticed herself "channeling" my way of relating, speaking in a more nurturing tone of voice and holding firmer boundaries. We decided to focus next on gently building Maisie's resilience to change and spontaneity.

SESSIONS 17–25

I intentionally stretched Maisie's need for sameness by altering some of our normal rituals. At first, Maisie struggled with this, withdrawing, but over a period of three sessions, she was able to emotionally navigate the increased flexibility in our routine. Providing her with words for her experience helped: "We're not doing it the same way today. You're not so sure it will still be fun."

I also began scaffolding Clarissa into a leadership role. At the beginning of this shift, Maisie became overly silly and made efforts to take control, but Clarissa responded with a confident, warm approach. Maisie regulated back to baseline with impressive speed. She fully trusted her mother to care for her needs and bring the fun.

Theraplay reduced Maisie's anxiety significantly. Now, during immunizations, she snuggled on her mother's lap and shed just a few tears. Maisie slept in her own bedroom with confidence every night, happily separated from her mother for school, and moved freely and independently throughout her home. She no longer suffered from panic attacks.

Conclusion

Anxiety disorders are prevalent, often intergenerational, and treatable. Anxiety can be mediated in childhood through building secure attachments and authoritative parenting practices; the most effective treatment models center on hand-over-hand guidance for caregivers. Structure—predictability and role definition—creates conditions in which both anxious children and caregivers can thrive.

Questions for reflection and continued learning

1. Can you name the two most important themes for Theraplay intervention with anxiety disorders? Generate three to five specific, play-based intervention ideas for each theme.

2. During a session, your child client resists structure by screaming at his mother. His mom anxiously withdraws, and while physically present for the rest of session, she seems shaken and distant. She emails you to cancel the next session with a vague reason. What is one strategy you might employ to prevent this scenario, and one strategy you might use in response to this situation?

3. Explore how you could meet an anxious caregiver's need for more contact between play sessions. Would you modify your between-session communication boundaries? Add caregiver sessions? Begin treatment with more caregiver-only work? Which modification(s) have full integrity for your professional values and your own self-care needs? Which modifications would generate resentment towards your clients or be lacking integrity for you as a practitioner? Why?

References

Baumrind, D. (1967). "Child care practices anteceding three patterns of preschool behavior." *Genetic Psychology Monographs, 75*(1), 43–88.

Booth, P.B. & Lindaman, S. (2010). *Understanding the Theory and Research that Inform the Core Concepts of Theraplay in Theraplay: Helping Parents and Children Build Better Relationships through Attachment-Based Play.* San Francisco, CA: Jossey-Bass.

Breinholst, S., Esbjørn, B.H., Reinholdt-Dunne, M.L. & Stallard, P. (2012). "CBT for the treatment of child anxiety disorders: A review of why parental involvement has not enhanced outcomes." *Journal of Anxiety Disorders, 26*(3), 416–424. Retrieved from https://doi.org/10.1016/j.janxdis.2011.12.014.

Colonnesi, C., Draijer, E.M., Stams, G.J., Van der Bruggen, C.O., Bögels, S.M. & Noom, M.J. (2011). "The relation between insecure attachment and child anxiety: A meta-analytic review." *Journal of Clinical Child & Adolescent Psychology, 40*(4), 630–645. doi:10.1080/15374416.2011.581623.

Costello, E., Mustillo, S., Erkani, A., Keeler, G. et al. (2003). "Prevalence and development of psychiatric disorders in childhood and adolescence." *Archives of General Psychiatry, 60,* 837–844.

Glibota, L.C., Lindaman, S. & Coleman, A.R. (2018). "Theraplay as a Treatment for Children with Selective Mutism: Integrating the Polyvagal Theory, Attachment Theory, and Social Communication." In A.A. Drewes & C. Schaefer (eds) *Play-Based Interventions for Childhood Anxieties, Fears and Phobias* (pp.124–143). New York, NY: Guilford Press.

Gregory, A.M. & Eley, T.C. (2007). "Genetic influences on anxiety in children: What we've learned and where we're heading." *Clinical Child and Family Psychology Review, 10*, 199–212.

Hibbard, D.R. & Walton, G.E. (2014). "Exploring the development of perfectionism: The influence of parenting style and gender." *Social Behavior and Personality: An International Journal, 42*(2), 269–278. Retrieved from https://doi.org/10.2224/sbp.2014.42.2.269.

Hudson, J.L. & Rapee, R.M. (2004). "From Anxious Temperament to Disorder: An Etiological Model of Generalized Anxiety Disorder." In R.G. Heimberg, C.L. Turk & D.S. Mennin (eds) *Generalized Anxiety Disorder: Advances in Research and Practice* (pp.51–76). New York, NY: Guilford Press.

Jacobvitz, D., Hazen, N., Curran, M. & Hitchens, K. (2004). "Observations of early triadic family interactions: Boundary disturbances in the family predict symptoms of depression, anxiety, and attention-deficit/hyperactivity disorder in middle childhood." *Development and Psychopathology, 16*(3), 577–592. doi:10.1017/S0954579404004675.

Katz, J., Petracca, M. & Rabinowitz, J. (2009). "A retrospective study of daughters' emotional role reversal with parents, attachment anxiety, excessive reassurance-seeking, and depressive symptoms." *American Journal of Family Therapy, 37*(3), 185–195.

Manassis, K., Lee, T.C., Bennett, K., Zhao, X.Y. *et al.* (2014). "Types of parental involvement in CBT with anxious youth: A preliminary meta-analysis." *Journal of Consulting and Clinical Psychology, 82*(6), 1163–1172. Retrieved from http://dx.doi.org/10.1037/a0036969.

McLeod, B.D., Wood, J.J. & Weisz, J.R. (2007). "Examining the association between parenting and childhood anxiety: A meta-analysis." *Clinical Psychology Review, 27*, 155–172.

Muris, P. & Field, A. (2013). "Information Processing Biases." In C.A. Essau & T.H. Ollendick (eds) *The Wiley-Blackwell Handbook of the Treatment of Childhood and Adolescent Anxiety* (pp.141–156). Chichester, UK: Wiley-Blackwell.

Paulussen-Hoogeboom, M.C., Stams, G.J., Hermanns, J.M., Peetsma, T.T. & van den Wittenboer, G.L. (2008). "Parenting style as a mediator between children's negative emotionality and problematic behavior in early childhood." *The Journal of Genetic Psychology, 169*(3), 209–226. doi:10.3200/GNTP.169.3.09-226.

Rapee, R.M., Schniering, C.A. & Hudson, J.L. (2009). "Anxiety disorders during childhood and adolescence: Origins and treatment." *Annual Review of Clinical Psychology, 5*, 311–341.

Rinaldia, C.M. & Howe, N. (2012). "Mothers' and fathers' parenting styles and associations with toddlers' externalizing, internalizing, and adaptive behaviors." *Early Childhood Research Quarterly, 27*(2), 266–273. Retrieved from https://doi.org/10.1016/j.ecresq.2011.08.001.

Rubin, K.H., Burgess, K.B. & Hastings, P.D. (2002). "Stability and social-behavioral consequences of toddlers' inhibited temperament and parenting behaviors." *Child Development, 73*(2), 483–495. doi:10.1111/1467-8624.00419.

Rubin, K.H., Coplan, R.J. & Bowker, J.C. (2009). "Social withdrawal in childhood." *Annual Review of Psychology, 60,* 141–171.

Schimmenti, A. & Bifulco, A. (2013). "Linking lack of care in childhood to anxiety disorders in emerging adulthood: The role of attachment styles." *Child & Adolescent Mental Health, 20,* 41–48. doi:10.1111/camh.12051.

Schniering, C.A. & Lyneham, H.J. (2007). "The Children's Automatic Thoughts Scale in a clinical sample: Psychometric properties and clinical utility." *Behaviour Research and Therapy, 45,* 1931–1940.

Schore, A.N. (2009). "Right-Brain Affect Regulation: An Essential Mechanism of Development, Trauma, Dissociation, and Psychotherapy." In D. Fosha, D.J. Siegel & M.F. Solomon (eds) *The Healing Power of Emotion: Affective Neuroscience, Development & Clinical Practice* (pp.112–144). New York, NY: W.W. Norton & Company.

Shamir-Essakow, G., Ungerer, J.A. & Rapee, R.M. (2005). "Attachment, behavioral inhibition, and anxiety in preschool children." *Journal of Abnormal Child Psychology, 33,* 131–143. Retrieved from https://doi.org/10.1007/s10802-005-1822-2.

Siu, A.F.Y. (2009). "Theraplay in the Chinese world: An intervention program for Hong Kong children with internalizing problems." *International Journal of Play Therapy, 18*(1), 1–12.

Tan, S., Moulding, R., Nedeljkovic, M. & Kyrios, M. (2010). "Metacognitive, cognitive and developmental predictors of generalised anxiety disorder symptoms." *Clinical Psychologist, 14*(3), 84–89. doi:10.1080/13284207.2010.521521.

Tucker, C., Schieffer, K., Wills, T., Hull, C. & Murphy, Q. (2017). "Enhancing social-emotional skills in at-risk preschool students through Theraplay based groups: The Sunshine Circle Model." *International Journal of Play Therapy, 26*(4), 185–195.

Van den Bergh, B.R.H., Mulder, E.J.H., Mennes, M. & Glover, V. (2005). "Antenatal maternal anxiety and stress and the neurobehavioural development of the fetus and child: Links and possible mechanisms, a review." *Neuroscience & Biobehavioral Reviews, 29*(2), 237–258. Retrieved from https://doi.org/10.1016/j.neubiorev.2004.10.007.

Wettig, H.G., Coleman, A.R. & Geider, F.J. (2011). "Evaluating the effectiveness of Theraplay in treating shy, socially withdrawn children." *International Journal of Play Therapy, 20*(1), 26–37.

Williams, K.E., Ciarrochi, J. & Heaven, P.C.L. (2012). "Inflexible parents, inflexible kids: A 6-year longitudinal study of parenting style and the development of psychological flexibility in adolescents." *Journal of Youth Adolescence, 41,* 1053–1066. Retrieved from https://doi.org/10.1007/s10964-012-9744-0.

Williams, L.R., Degnan, K.A., Perez-Edgar, K.E., Henderson, H.A. *et al.* (2009). "Impact of behavioral inhibition and parenting style on internalizing and externalizing problems from early childhood through adolescence." *Journal of Abnormal Child Psychology, 37*(8), 1063–1075.

Chapter 8

Using Theraplay to Treat Clients of Child Sexual Abuse

Elizabeth Konrath and Eliana Gil

Introduction

This chapter will specify why and how Theraplay is a valuable treatment when working with sexually abused children. Most child sexual abuse (CSA) occurs in the context of an important relationship, whether a family member or other trusted older child or adult. In addition, child sexual abuse affects the relationship with the non-offending caregiver as well, often causing a range of feelings, including isolation, confusion, shame and fear. Sexual abuse exposes children to inappropriate boundaries, role-reversals in which their needs are secondary, and expectations of secrecy. The abuser sets aside their victim's developmental needs and expects the child to behave as a partner in complex interpersonal dynamics. The child is seduced into believing that they are having a "special" loving relationship and yet they have conflictual parallel feelings and develop inaccurate perceptions and thoughts about the type and amount of special attention they receive. The experience of physical touch becomes perplexing and complex: children may feel exposed, vulnerable, even embarrassed, and yet may have some pleasurable sensations in their bodies. Sexually abused children also are exposed to individuals who act one way with them in private and another way in public. This makes it difficult to understand boundaries, physical affection, sensual or sexual experiences, along with a host of varied and idiosyncratic feelings and thoughts.

The children also face challenges with peer relationships and self-imposed isolation. Finally, research shows that sexually abused children typically have difficulties with attachment, biology, physical and behavioral dysregulation, self-esteem and dissociation (National Child Traumatic Stress Network, 2019).

Key points

Theraplay provides the following therapeutic responses to address the trauma variables described above:

1. Developing emotional and behavioral regulation and co-regulation to combat feelings of fear, confusion and shame.

2. Establishing or re-establishing a more secure attachment in order to reduce feelings of isolation, and to correct role reversals and distortions about the nature of adult-child relationships.

3. Creating relational boundaries, including the safe and healthy use of touch in order to emphasize the child's needs for touch rather than the adult's needs.

4. Prioritizing the child's developmental needs so that the child feels seen, heard and understood through play, rather than verbal interactions relating to the abuse.

5. Encouraging mastery and control to improve self-esteem and build empowerment.

6. Focusing on the here and now, which can protect against dissociative responses.

Theraplay-based treatment goals for the above as well as other target areas will be discussed in detail in this chapter.

Significance of the topic

An increasing number of mental health professionals, including Theraplay specialists, receive referrals specific to child sexual abuse. Although other evidence-based treatments may be prioritized for children who have experienced sexual abuse, Theraplay is a valuable treatment option, particularly since it supports the child and their family relationships and targets many of the treatment goals considered relevant for this population. We will discuss the ways to use Theraplay as an intervention in conjunction with other modalities when working with children who have suffered sexual abuse. We will also explore when to use Theraplay in treatment, as it may be appropriate to use Theraplay either prior to the trauma processing, or after trauma-focused therapy has occurred.

Child sexual abuse is a uniquely complex and challenging issue for mental health professionals to manage and treat. It is crucial that practitioners who are working with children who have been sexually abused are well trained in issues related to childhood trauma and child maltreatment and have substantial experience in Theraplay as well as other trauma-focused modalities. Child sexual abuse is rarely a discrete event, and it typically occurs in a larger context of neglect or other family dysfunction. Therefore, this chapter is focused on treating child sexual abuse not as a single occurrence, but rather occurring alongside other dysfunctional patterns.

Background information

Child sexual abuse is defined as "any interaction between a child and an adult (or another child) in which the child is used for the sexual stimulation of the perpetrator or observer" (National Child Traumatic Stress Network, 2019). Sexual abuse can include behaviors where the child is touched, but it can also include non-touching behaviors, such as voyeurism, exposing a child to pornography, or exhibitionism (National Child Traumatic Stress Network, 2019). CSA is not limited to children of specific ages, races, ethnicities and economic backgrounds, as any child from any community may experience sexual abuse. The statistics on child sexual abuse are jarring and saddening. Studies reveal that one in five girls and one in 20 boys is a victim of child sexual abuse, and 28 percent of young people aged 14–17 have been sexually victimized in the United States (Finkelhor, 2009). Furthermore, according to several sources, between 75 and 93 percent of adolescents who were sexually abused were victimized by someone they knew well or by a family member (Finkelhor *et al.*, 2014).

Research over the past several decades confirms that child sexual abuse has profound long-term effects on the victim. It has been linked to higher levels of depression, guilt, shame, self-blame, eating disorders, sleep disruptions, anxiety, dissociation, relationship problems and mood disorders (Felitti *et al.*, 2019). The Adverse Childhood Experiences (ACE)

Study found that exposure to traumatic experiences in childhood is strongly associated with health risk behavior and disease in adulthood, including alcoholism, drug abuse, heart disease and other health problems (Felitti *et al.*, 2019). Individuals who have suffered sexual abuse as a child are more likely to experience post-traumatic stress disorder, which can have a detrimental impact on the neurobiological functioning and development of a child (Hodges *et al.*, 2013). Additionally, CSA can have an impact on future relationships and functioning. ACE studies have linked CSA to a higher risk of experiencing sexual victimization in adulthood (Ports, Ford & Merrick, 2016).

The individual victim is not the only person to suffer as a result of child sexual abuse—the familial relationships and attachment bonds are severely impacted by this abuse. Caregivers have reported feelings of guilt, anxiety, fear and emotional stress due to the sexual abuse of their child (Karakurt & Silver, 2014).

Current treatment trends

The National Child Traumatic Stress Network (NCTSN) is a current, reliable resource that provides state-of-the art information and training, supports empirical studies and holds an unrivaled leadership role in the field of childhood trauma. NCTSN has reviewed major treatment interventions and developed a consensus of target-affected areas and treatment goals for this population. These targeted areas include: attachment, biology, behavioral and emotional regulation, dissociation and self-esteem. Van der Kolk (2015) describes six core components for treatment that include prioritizing safety, self-regulation, self-reflective information processing, integration of traumatic experiences, relational engagement and positive affect enhancement (discussed later in this chapter). Perry suggests that positive treatment experiences must be relational, relevant, repetitive, rewarding, rhythmic and respectful (Perry, 2006).

Although there is general agreement on the assessment and treatment components and goals when working with sexually abused children, treatment approaches remain varied but definitively more trauma-informed than ever. NCTSN has singled out three primary evidence-based treatments that have been shown to be effective in improving trauma-specific outcomes for children who have experienced abuse. These treatments are:

1. problematic sexual-behavior-cognitive behavioral therapy for school-age children

2. risk reduction through family therapy

3. trauma-focused cognitive behavioral therapy (TF-CBT).

It is important to note that all the recommended interventions for CSA involve the family in treatment. All three of these models are found to be beneficial for families of diverse racial and cultural backgrounds, although most of the research on the efficacy has been conducted in the United States.

Recent advances in the study of neuroscience have contributed greatly to our understanding of the impact of adverse childhood experiences and helped us consider how best to deliver treatment services to young children. The Child Trauma Academy (CTA) and Bruce Perry have developed an approach to treating children with complex trauma called the Neurosequential Model of Therapeutics (NMT). NMT assesses a child's strengths, vulnerabilities, history and development, and then determines the approaches to best meet the client's needs (Gaskill & Perry, 2013). Perry's model does not single out treatment approaches, but rather the focus and timing of treatment delivery. Perry has stated that cognitive interventions (such as TF-CBT) might best be delivered after the child's regulatory system has been soothed and their relationships have been secured.

Stephen Porges' polyvagal theory (2011), a recent development in the field of neuroscience, provides clinicians with a deeper understanding of safety in working with clients who have experienced complex trauma. This theory explains a part of the nervous system that had been previously overlooked, which Porges refers to as the "social engagement system." The social engagement system is responsible for navigating relationships and for activating higher brain functions, such as playfulness, intimacy and creativity, but it cannot be accessed unless one experiences safety and trust. Polyvagal theory explains the connection between what happens in one's body and how that influences one's feelings and behaviors, which then impacts one's relationships and ability to interact with others. Porges explores the ways that psychiatric health problems are the result of failures of reciprocal social engagement in relationships.

Van der Kolk, in his book *The Body Keeps the Score* (2015), emphasizes the need for treatment to expand into visceral, sensory and physical dimensions. He questions the reliance on talk therapy and highlights the value of integrating multiple modalities, particularly those that incorporate movement and pleasure to build regulation. Attachment, regulation and competency (ARC) is an evidence-based, trauma-informed treatment model that focuses on four primary areas: typical childhood development, traumatic stress, attachment and risk/resilience (Blaustein & Kinniburgh, 2018). At the foundation of the ARC model is the knowledge that without first building a safe attachment system, all the other developmental competencies cannot be established (Arvidson *et al.*, 2011). Another therapeutic model that emphasizes the body-brain connection is sensorimotor psychotherapy, developed by Pat Ogden (Lohrasbe & Ogden, 2017). At the basis of sensorimotor psychotherapy is the knowledge that trauma has a profound impact on the body, and the symptoms are somatically based. Sensorimotor psychotherapy first works to treat the impact of the trauma on the body, before focusing on cognitive/emotional processing (Lohrasbe & Ogden, 2017). These several beneficial approaches to treating trauma clearly indicate that ethical and relevant treatment must be an integrated approach that focuses on a "bottom-up" approach, including strategies to address symptoms in both the brain and body.

Support for Theraplay in the treatment of child sexual abuse

There is a strong clinical context and rationale for using Theraplay as an adjunctive modality to help children heal from sexual abuse, and numerous benefits to using Theraplay while treating sexually abused children. Kezelman and Stavropoulos (2012) recognize a three-phased approach to successfully treating CSA, including: promoting safety and security, processing the trauma, and integrating and moving forward.

Traditionally, mental health professionals working with child sexual abuse have been ambivalent about introducing touch into the therapy session. Experienced sexual abuse providers have cautioned that children may bring up sexual themes in their play, may cross physical boundaries with therapists, or may re-enact victim/victimizer dynamics in their play, often utilizing a unique expression defined as post-traumatic play (Gil, 2017). In addition, mental health professionals working with sexually abused children have favored an individual approach with collateral dyadic parent-child sessions later in treatment. Theraplay, with its deliberate use of touch, its interactive play and its inclusion of parents in sessions, is clearly a different approach. The following six areas explore the benefits and special considerations for using Theraplay when working with children who have been sexually abused.

1. Development of emotional and behavioral regulation and co-regulation

Data from neuroscience resonates with the Theraplay model. As Gaskill and Perry (2013) suggest, effective treatment must address the physical needs of the child's nervous system. Theraplay offers "bottom-up" techniques that focus on the brain stem's regulatory and physiological systems (such as pulse and heart rate, activated by stress). Theraplay activities are whole-brain approaches that promote vertical (body and mind) and horizontal (left and right hemispheres) communication in the brain, so that children build better emotional and physical regulation. Co-regulation within a secure relationship is a useful and critical sign of relational health. Because the Theraplay model includes a caregiver/parent directly in the sessions, it allows the caregiver to learn to become an external co-regulator for the child. Theraplay helps children achieve healthy and positive ways of thinking, feeling and behaving. It is a therapeutic model that is designed to restore feelings of safety in the here and now within a relational context. Thus, safety, trust and attachment are simultaneously supported utilizing Theraplay.

The following is an example of how the Theraplay practitioner creates moments of co-regulation during a Theraplay session. The practitioner introduces a mirroring game, where the child copies the physical movements and facial expressions of the therapist as if looking directly into a mirror. During this activity, the practitioner is providing structure, while also maintaining attunement to the child. Based on the child's arousal level, the practitioner can moderate the amount of energy, movement and physical proximity to the child. The practitioner may start by taking steps forward and backward from the child, moving slowly or quickly, stomping feet on the ground, doing deep breathing or stretching up to the sky, all depending on the child's need for physical regulation.

2. Re-establishment of feelings of safety and a secure attachment

Relational interventions have been found to be pivotal to success whether or not the child has been sexually abused within the family. Children cannot be treated in isolation from their important relationships, and thus child sexual abuse is a systemic issue that warrants a systemic response (Gil, 2006). Sheinberg and Fraenkel (2001) state that sexual abuse of a child can violate the entire family system's sense of security and disrupts the attachments between family members. Relationships may feel different with each parent and sibling, and the security and predictability of parent-child relationships may be in question. Because of this, Sheinberg and Fraenkel emphasize the benefits of working within the family system in order to strengthen safe attachment relationships and help families create a secure base for the children and the non-offending adults.

The Theraplay model is a preverbal approach to healing and it directly addresses safety in the relationship to prepare the child to process the trauma. Theraplay is designed to pursue changes in attachment in a direct way, creating or rebuilding a secure attachment for the caregiver and child—with sexually abused children in particular, secure attachments are linked to successful treatment outcomes.

As noted earlier, child sexual abuse typically occurs in a larger context of neglect or other type of family dysfunction. The practitioner uses the assessment interviews, the interaction observation, reflective discussion and parent practice to learn about the family function as well as the impact of the abuse and to develop trust and attunement with the caregiver. Prior to starting dyadic Theraplay sessions, the practitioner must consider the capacity of the caregiver to follow directives and provide appropriate responses to their children. The practitioner must determine if the caregiver harbors resentment or anger towards the child and consequently is not prioritizing the child's needs for safety and protection. As with any other caregiver, one who is actively abusing the child, using drugs or alcohol or is not capable of a healthy attachment should not be included in Theraplay sessions, and other modalities should be considered.

In the standard Theraplay protocol, a caregiver is typically in the room right from the beginning, observing while the practitioner establishes routines and builds a relationship with the child. For the child with CSA, the presence of the caregiver in the room builds the child's sense of safety with the practitioner. This is particularly true for a child who was isolated or alone with an adult when the sexual abuse occurred (Rubin, Lender & Mroz-Miller, 2010). Since there is typically no talk about the abuse during the weekly sessions, the child may feel less self-protective and more fully engaged and ready to play with the caregiver. When working with children who have been sexually abused, the caregiver often is asked to help the practitioner from the outset. When the practitioner demonstrates an activity with the caregiver rather than directly with the child, it helps the child understand what will happen so that it is more likely the child will feel safe. For instance, if a practitioner plans to make a handprint of the child's hand, the practitioner will need to be highly attuned to the child and read their non-verbal communication. If the child's face is not curious, but rather appears afraid, if they physically move away, or even refuse to do the activity, the practitioner can instead do the activity with the caregiver first. The practitioner might enlist the child to help put lotion on the caregiver's hand, push it gently down on the paper, and then hold the paper while the practitioner sprinkles baby powder on it to see the print. Often when the child observes the caregiver doing the activity and knows what to expect, they will feel safer and more open to participating.

As a caregiver participates in the sessions and works to build a safe and secure relationship with the child, they are communicating that they are safe and present for their child. Each activity is designed to provide the caregiver with the experience of attuning to, accepting and supporting their child. For example, a child who is feeling overwhelmed at some point in the session might hide their face in a pillow. The therapist then turns this into an activity where the child and the caregiver hide together so the child does not feel isolated and can remain connected with the caregiver (and vice versa). Then the practitioner can "find" them in the room three different times, each time delighting in finding them together, making eye contact and connecting with the child after the short break of hiding.

Sometimes, a practitioner senses that the child does not believe that the caregiver can maintain these interactions with them outside the sessions. In this situation, the practitioner should discuss this possibility with the caregiver and then acknowledge it in a session. A practitioner might say "You're not sure your mom can keep this up outside this office" or "You're not totally sure your mom can keep you safe. Is that right?" The dyad will benefit from hearing the practitioner and caregiver validate this concern for the child and reiterate that, even though it sometimes may be hard, the caregiver desires to and intends to maintain the safety and interaction of the Theraplay sessions outside therapy.

3. Establishment of relational boundaries, including safe and healthy use of touch

Theraplay practitioners clarify physical boundaries for both the child and caregivers and provide healthy interpersonal interactions that include the safe, reparative touch that is so crucial for children who have experienced sexual abuse. Child sexual abuse typically disrupts the child's feelings of safety and, as mentioned previously, can create negative feelings of self-worth. Theraplay practitioners can help children re-establish an accurate sense of who they are and what their strengths are, and teach them to expect that their developmental needs will be met. Thus, children can reorder their narratives to pre-abuse functioning of safety, virtue and positive identity if such existed, or they can build a more balanced, positive narrative. Building self-esteem and positive self-worth can also be protective factors in decreasing a child's risk of being sexually abused in the future (Wilcox, Richards & O'Keefe, 2004).

Ways to incorporate healthy and safe touch in a Theraplay session include activities that utilize both the structure and nurture dimensions. For instance, taking a foil print of a child's hands, elbows, feet or knees provides the child with structuring touch throughout the activity, and with less opportunity for confusion about the touch. The practitioner facilitates the interaction between the caregiver and the child so that, through this activity, they are both experiencing the different body parts with delight (i.e., "Look how big your feet are growing!" or "Wow, this is a very pointy elbow your child has here, Dad!").

Rubin and colleagues (2010) find it imperative to be clear about boundaries. In some instances, it is important for the caregiver to inform the child before the first session that the practitioner they are going to see does indeed know about the sexual abuse. Then in the session, the practitioner will need to state that he or she knows what happened to the child and why they are in treatment. After asking the child what their understanding is of why they are coming to therapy, the practitioner should clarify that the treatment is related to the allegation or occurrence of child sexual abuse. A practitioner can make statements such as "I heard from your mom that your brother touched your private parts" or "Your father told me that your teacher was touching your private parts and telling you it was your secret game." It will be relevant for the practitioner to describe what will and will not happen in treatment. Of course, because children have had relational injuries, practitioners can add, "You will not be hit or hurt in this office and there will not be touching of private parts. I may remind you of this as we get to know each other better." A practitioner will need to communicate these messages in a consistent manner that will not overwhelm the child; for instance, pausing, reacting to the child's response, and reading their non-verbal cues. The purpose of these statements is to reassure the child from the very beginning, so that they do not feel confused or anxious about what may happen in session or about the purpose of therapy. Such statements will need to be restated throughout treatment, not just in the initial stages. This is particularly salient for sexually abused children who may feel confused if they have experienced playfulness and intimacy from an adult as a part of a seductive interaction which led to abuse.

Sexually abused children may develop a fear of touching or being touched by others or may have learned inappropriate physical boundaries that are activated in different situations or with specific people. In addition, practitioners may feel afraid of triggering or confusing children, so they maintain rigid physical boundaries, which also sends confusing messages to the child. Theraplay activities are designed to help children learn about healthy and safe, structured and nurturing touch that they need and deserve for healthy growth. Using touch in sessions with a child who has been sexually abused needs to be matter of fact, non-intrusive and non-threatening (Rubin *et al.*, 2010). Children who experience sexual abuse are commonly taught that their bodies are special for what they provide to the abuser. Through the use of the Theraplay model of treatment, children learn that there are many unique and special things about them and their bodies that have nothing to do with sex or being hurt.

Sexually abused children can become confused about boundaries, adult intention and their bodies during a session, and these feelings can cause acting-out behaviors. Theraplay practitioners should anticipate some of the causes of sexualized behavior and develop very specific physical and verbal responses. Therapeutic responses should be calm, non-judgmental and clear. Recording the sessions can help clinicians identify what may have elicited sexual behaviors from the child in the session. Because caregivers might not feel comfortable or confident setting limits or responding in the moment to their child's sexual acting out, it is helpful to speak with the caregiver without the child present if this happens so that the therapist can model and process for the caregiver how to respond to such behaviors outside the office.

4. Prioritization of children's developmental needs

Abusers place demands on children that far exceed their developmental capacities. Thus, at a time when children should be carefree, curious, playful and cared for, they are instead required to keep secrets, negotiate adult needs and, most importantly, negotiate them alone. Typically, children's caregivers are their most important resource, but in familial sexual abuse, the abusive person seeks compliance about secrecy, specifying the abuse as a special bond that must be protected. Thus, children are left alone to figure out what to do and are often afraid to disclose the abuse verbally to other adults.

Play is the universal language of children. It is how they communicate, learn and practice new skills and regulate themselves physically and emotionally, and how they connect to others. Because the Theraplay model is play based, it works efficiently to meet these goals while being developmentally appropriate for a child. In the bean-bag drop activity the child has the opportunity to participate in a back-and-forth, face-to-face, engaging activity that ends with the success of catching the bean bag. The practitioner places the bean bag on her own head and gives a "signal" (a cue word or a facial signal such as a nose wiggle, eyebrow raise or eye blink) before dropping it in the child's hands. This simple activity communicates a number of different and important messages to the child: *I see you, I am here with you, I delight in you, I am paying attention to you.*

Another benefit of using Theraplay with sexually abused children is that the model does not rely on verbal interactions. Disclosures for children and families can create tension, confusion and conflict. Children may have had to disclose their abuse over and over to various different people. By the time they come to therapy, the last thing they want to do is talk about what happened to them. Theraplay practitioners provide treatment and meet therapeutic goals without focusing on talking, thus being developmentally attuned to a child's needs. Theraplay helps both the child and caregiver fine-tune their interactions, returning to an earlier time when the child communicated without words and the caregivers developed responses based on attunement. The child feels seen, heard and understood in their earlier language, that of play, behavior and non-verbal expression.

5. Encouragement of mastery and control

Sexual abuse is not exclusively about sex for either child or abuser. Most sex offenders appear to be seeking power and control over their victims. Therefore, children who have been sexually abused need and benefit from opportunities to experience the world from a place of empowerment. Practitioners can provide many decision-making and mastery opportunities for abused children so they can directly disconfirm their sense of vulnerability and helplessness. The structured choices that practitioners provide throughout Theraplay sessions—such as asking, "Do you want the red balloon or the yellow balloon?"—help children experience autonomy without putting pressure on them to be in control. Activities within the challenge dimension also are helpful to improve a child's self-esteem and gain feelings of empowerment and pride in themselves. For example, in balloon volleyball, the practitioner, child and caregiver see how many hits between them they can do to keep the balloon up in the air. As they play, the practitioner exclaims, "Wow, nice save! Your arms are so strong! You're so focused on hitting these balloons straight to me!" In this example, the child is being given an opportunity to engage in an activity that is difficult, but not impossible or discouraging. Both the child and the caregiver are experiencing the child's body as strong and capable, while also engaging in a joyful, pleasurable interaction.

6. Focus on the here and now

Theraplay is a physically active therapy approach that happens in vivo between practitioner, caregiver and child. A child who has been sexually abused may have developed defense systems that are unhealthy or maladaptive. Dissociation, commonly associated with trauma, is a key example. Dissociation is an important defense that clinicians must learn to recognize (Silberg, 2013). During dissociation, which can be activated at any time and via any known or unknown triggers during therapy, children seek to "leave the experience" by having out-of-body experiences. This disintegrative defense can produce alterations in the child's identity, consciousness and memory. Thus, the child might question if the experience happened to them directly or someone else, and their memories might feel dream-like. A practitioner must recognize the importance of the child's initial need for self-protection. A child will not, and should not, be encouraged to abandon those defenses until they have replaced them with healthy protective mechanisms. The Theraplay practitioner will need to find a balance between providing structure and allowing the child to feel empowered and in control. For example, a child who may be feeling overwhelmed by the session activities might simply pull away, sit down or face a corner of the room. They also may just look at a spot on the wall and get very still. The practitioner can observe this behavior, leave it for a few minutes, and then gradually introduce a non-threatening activity such as blowing bubbles, allowing them to fall on the ground in front of the child. When the child reorients to the room, the practitioner can instruct the child to pop the bubbles and slowly become interactive again.

Theraplay practitioners encourage the child to stay in the present to experience the physical, engaging, challenging or nurturing interactions available to them at this moment. The focus in Theraplay is on the establishment of safety and trust. As children feel safer and more trusting, there is less need for dissociative responses.

In summary, Theraplay treatment can work directly with target treatment issues typically found in sexually abused children and their families. Theraplay is uniquely suited for this work because it prioritizes secure attachment, regulation, boundary-setting and the developmental needs of the child, strengthens caregiver capacities for providing components of healthy attachment and gives the caregiver and child opportunities to restore a sense of mastery and control. Theraplay is best viewed either as an adjunctive therapy that can be provided early on to help children regulate enough to do trauma work, or later, once the trauma work is done, when caregivers are ready to refocus on their children's needs, and the caregiver-child relationship is ready for a structured approach to re-establish or strengthen secure attachment. Theraplay is delivered in a lively, physical, engaging way that promotes relational pleasure and joy and helps children reconnect safely with their bodies.

CASE ILLUSTRATION

Eight-year-old Steven was referred to me (Elizabeth Konrath) specifically for Theraplay services. His mother, Jennifer, and I spoke on the phone briefly so that I could provide her with some basic information about the therapy process and she could discuss her concerns. She had three other children who were currently working with therapists in another practice, so she was well versed in the therapy process. She shared very little about Steven on the phone except that he and all his siblings had been sexually abused for many years by a babysitter.

I was surprised to find Steven in the waiting room when I went to greet Jennifer for our intake appointment. She had brought Steven with her because the babysitter had cancelled before the appointment. Steven was a small, energetic child, with bright eyes and a huge smile. Because I knew that he had been a victim of trauma, I felt it was important for him to be comfortable in his surroundings. I took extra time to engage with him, walk him around the office suite, giving him an explanation of the different rooms, the other therapists working in the suite, the kitchen area, restrooms and the room in which his mother and I would be meeting. Although I gave Steven an array of books and coloring supplies, my meeting with Jennifer was peppered with his interruptions. He was understandably concerned about what information his mother was sharing about him, and his anxiety increased throughout the hour. He repeatedly came into the room, disrupting the intake so many times we opted to reschedule. Steven asked me, "Are you going to take me away from my mommy?"—which confused me until Jennifer explained, in front of Steven, that she was considering residential treatment for him, and that this therapy was his "last shot." I knelt down and looked directly at Steven, my hand on his shoulder. "Actually, my job is to work very, very hard to help you and your mommy stay together. I don't take kids away from their parents, but I try to help them be a better team and feel better with each other."

In the subsequent intake meeting, Jennifer provided more in-depth information about Steven's history, including that he had been removed from her care the first two years of his life due to substantiated findings of neglect. Jennifer was reunited with Steven after meeting court requirements for steady income and housing and now cared for him and his three younger siblings as a working single mother. She had relied on a 14-year-old neighbor boy, Neal, to watch her four children after school.

Jennifer teared up as she described how Steven would beg her not to leave and would scream in the mornings before Jennifer took him to school because Neal would be there after school to watch them. She reflected that she "should have known" what was happening, but did not recognize signs that Neal was sexually abusing the children for years. There were, however, very concerning and obvious signs, including disclosures that Jennifer did not believe. Finally, one of Steven's younger brothers disclosed the abuse to a teacher at school, who called Child Protective Services. They launched a full investigation, arrested Neal, and ordered each child into therapy.

Jennifer described how Steven had "always" been a challenging child even as a baby, but his behaviors in the past two years had become totally unmanageable. She described Steven's impulsivity and stated that he ran from her in public places and darted into traffic. He also had difficulty focusing and sitting still as well as very long, drawn-out screaming and raging tantrums, almost daily. Jennifer confided two things to me: that she felt helpless and exhausted and did not want to be around Steven anymore, and that she was consumed by guilt for not recognizing the sexual abuse and felt like an utter failure as a mother.

THERAPLAY PROCESS AND PROGRESSION

The MIM assessment between Steven and Jennifer, not surprisingly, revealed a number of challenges experienced by the dyad. Jennifer had a very difficult time engaging with Steven. He showed aggressive and rejecting behaviors towards Jennifer, and she appeared afraid to touch him or even sit near him. They hardly made any eye contact and appeared totally disconnected throughout the assessment. Steven refused any of his mother's attempts to set structure, laughing at her while doing the opposite of what she had requested, often stating, "I can do what I want and you won't do anything about it." Steven also refused to attempt new activities (challenge dimension) even as Jennifer encouraged or praised him.

When I came into the room at the end of the MIM to ask them questions, Jennifer stated to me, in front of Steven, "Well, that was awful. Just awful." In reviewing the MIM, there were indeed a number of difficult interactions, but I also found several examples of ways Jennifer was nurturing and soothing with Steven. I noted times when it appeared that Jennifer wanted to be more soothing and affectionate with Steven but seemed to hold back. I isolated these clips during my feedback session with her to emphasize her strengths, and she broke down crying. She stated that her friends and family members had advised her not to touch him, since it was likely that he associated any touch as inappropriate or harmful after the sexual abuse he had endured. She indicated she understood that logic, but felt very confused because it went against her instinct as a mother. She saw through clips in the MIM that her caution to provide him with physical touch created more distance from him and increased his dysregulation.

Before the feedback session, I already believed Theraplay was going to be the most effective way I could meet the treatment goals of regulating Steven, building their relationship, and giving Jennifer real-time, hands-on skills and coaching. But I also realized then that Theraplay would be the best way for me to help strengthen Jennifer's self-esteem as a mother and build her own confidence in her ability to relate to and support Steven. Although I felt totally overwhelmed and seriously considered referring the case to another therapist, I took some deep breaths, scheduled pre-emptively with my supervisor, and plunged into treatment.

The initial four or five Theraplay sessions started out with Steven running around the room wildly, sometimes even going into other therapists' offices to hide, or to disrupt their sessions. He would take my small bag of Theraplay items and throw it around the room, snatching my index card with the activities I'd planned for that session and hiding it, or ripping it up. I got very skilled at memorizing the activities I'd planned for Steven, as well as using fewer supplies throughout the sessions. I also worked to keep him physically contained, by sitting him on a bean bag, using my body to stop him from being able to run around, and holding his hand if he did get up, so that we remained physically connected. I also jumped right into activities very quickly, because if I ever took too long to verbally explain them, he would use that as an opportunity to get up and run around. As long as the transitions were quick, he would participate and learn that he enjoyed what I had planned. His mother attended every session from the beginning. I had instructed her to sit directly next to Steven and I asked her to try to allow me to respond to his behaviors without her intervening. Jennifer appeared to be quite overwhelmed and disengaged from sessions during that time, often moving away from us, sitting to the side, looking at her cell phone, or not responding to my efforts to include her in the activities.

Several times at the beginning of treatment, Steven would say to me, "You want me to talk about Neal and I'm not going to." I would assure Steven that even though I knew what Neal had done to him, right now Steven and I were not going to talk about that. I reiterated that we were going to spend some time getting to know and trust each other by playing together, and that I wanted to help him feel safe and calm in his body. In our early sessions, I emphasized activities in the structure dimension in order to build a sense of safety and predictability in our relationship. Almost all of the activities I chose involved us sitting on the floor, since when we stood up to do an activity, Steven ran around the room, and I would lose the engagement and connection.

SAMPLE SESSION OUTLINE OF ACTIVITIES

- Entrance: Structure/Engagement (counting how many big steps he could take from the door to the bean bag).

- Check-ups: Engagement/Nurture (noticing strong muscles, counting fingers and freckles on hands, measuring hands, feet, arms to see how big they're getting, caring for any hurts).

- Bean-bag drop: Engagement/Structure.

- Pass a sound: Engagement/Structure.

- Bubble pop: Engagement/Structure.

- Hide and seek: Engagement/Structure (Steven and Jennifer hide together, I find them).

- Cotton ball hockey: Engagement/Challenge.

- Blanket swing/Sing Twinkle Song: Nurture.

- Feeding: Nurture.

- Exit: Magic carpet ride: Structure/Engagement.

PROGRESSION AND OUTCOME

As therapy progressed, Steven became far more regulated. We established a routine in the sessions, and he became increasingly eager to engage with me, learn new activities, and actually even sat still for the bulk of the sessions. This was an indication that he was less hyperaroused, calmer and more organized physically. Steven became increasingly accepting and comfortable with me leading activities and setting limits, and would often say, "You're always the boss in here but it's still kind of fun." I would reply, "That's true! When I lead, we still have fun together. I'm really trying to pay attention to the games that you like." He frequently attempted to extend activities, despite my warning that it was our last time playing that particular game. He would say, "One more time! I want to do it again!" I would explain to him that it was our last time, but I would also make a note on the notecard that he really enjoyed that game and I would be sure we would repeat it in the next session.

He grew to enjoy the nurturing activities very much, requesting that they go on for longer and longer. Once when I was doing a weather report on his back (a massage that provides slow or fast manual motions depending on what season you are describing verbally), in an attempt to extend the activity, he stated, "You need to do all the seasons...spring, summer, fall and winter!"

At one point, after a weather report, Steven began to touch his penis through his pants. Admittedly, I was caught off guard and said to him, "Oh, I'm sorry, I should have told you, you don't ever have to do that in here," and then promptly moved on to a different activity. I showed my supervisor the recording of this session and she helped me figure out what to say if Steven did this again. I also spoke with Jennifer about this incident, and she said that he engaged in behaviors like this at home regularly. In the next session, Steven did almost exactly the same thing. As he started to touch himself again, I quickly stopped what I was doing and took his hands in mine. Then I said, "Oh my goodness! Steven, I am so sorry! I think that maybe when we were playing that game I confused you. I think that maybe someone taught you to do things like that with your body when they were playing with you. I did not realize when I did that, it might confuse you or make you feel that way. I will never ask you to do that with your body. I will never touch your private parts." Steven stared at me silently, not speaking. I wanted to stay engaged with him, and since I was holding his hands, we began doing a hand stack. I was careful to note the connection between the presence of these behaviors immediately following a nurturing activity, and I wondered if he confused my care and touch as grooming he had received from Neal just before he sexually abused Steven. He did not demonstrate these specific behaviors with me again in treatment, although he did often continue to push physical boundaries with me. I remained cautious and deliberate when using structuring and grounding touch in my work with Steven throughout therapy.

Jennifer continued to attend each session, and as Steven's behavior improved and he became more open to Theraplay, so did she. I met with her twice a month individually to review videos and explore Steven's reactions to the activities to help her gain more information and empathy about his behaviors. I also referred Jennifer to participate in the Circle of Security program (Powell *et al.*, 2016) with a colleague. Over time, Jennifer began to experience Steven in delightful ways rather than interacting with him in a corrective or punitive manner. She often smiled at him, engaged in genuine laughter when he was successful at activities, sat physically much closer to him, and often held his hand or put her arm around him. She gained skills and understanding in how to connect and co-regulate through the parenting sessions with me, Circle of Security, and the Theraplay sessions with Steven. Jennifer could consistently laugh, play and experience joy-filled interactions with her son, and he began to trust her as a safe haven again.

Jennifer thrived as she learned to interact in a nurturing way with her son. She learned that the physical affection that she was afraid to offer to Steven in the past was what he desperately needed to feel loved, cared for and regulated. The most difficult dimension of their relationship was limit-setting and providing him with structure. He continued to run away from her, yell at her, or throw a tantrum when she set limits. However, over time, she took a more obvious leadership role in Theraplay sessions and this translated into more successful moments of Steven following without resistance. Jennifer stated that she would "channel her Inner Lizzie" to set firm and consistent limits with Steven and her other children at home, and her confidence grew.

As noted in the Theraplay protocol, complex situations of trauma require a longer treatment period. After about ten months of weekly Theraplay, Steven showed marked improvement in his regulation and sense of safety, particularly in his relationship with his mother. Jennifer's skills of co-regulation, attunement and leadership had improved tremendously. At this point, I decided it was time to move to a more integrated approach for therapy to process Steven's trauma using Eliana Gil's trauma-focused integrated play therapy (TF-IPT) approach

(Gil, 2012). Because of the Theraplay sessions, Steven was regulated and secure enough to process the trauma both individually and with Jennifer as a supportive witness using the TF-IPT model.

Conclusion

The case illustrates the complexities of treating child sexual abuse, including the attachment disruption that occurs when a child has to negotiate the demands of sexual abuse alone. In this case, the child's emotional and behavioral dysregulation, attachment disruption, low self-esteem and feelings of isolation created havoc in his home, so much so that his exhausted mother was ready to find an out-of-home placement for him. This case was further exacerbated by the fact that the child had been removed from his mother for his first two years of life, due to neglect. His mother had fought hard to get him back and was trying hard to provide good care for him when his sexual abuse by a trusted babysitter began and continued for years, even as the child tried desperately to elicit his mother's protection.

Theraplay helped the mother-child dyad by allowing them to experience joint pleasure, by restoring a sense of trust, and by allowing the child to get his nurturing needs met by his mother. Steven's mother's confidence grew about her limit-setting capacities and co-regulation. Subsequently, the mother-child dyad engaged in trauma-focused therapy, which included cognitive-behavioral work. This case demonstrates how Perry's emphasis on treatment sequencing was of utmost importance.

More recent data from the neuroscientific field also provides a compelling case for alternative forms of therapy, including massage, yoga, animal-assisted therapy, music, movement, play, art and other forms of expressive therapies. In fact, most trauma-specific treatment programs are advocating for a broad range of approaches to augment verbal and cognitive therapies.

The Theraplay approach can be appropriate and necessary in cases of child sexual abuse, especially those in which the child's secure attachment has been disrupted by the caretaker's inability or unwillingness to take a protective stance for their child. As described at the outset, research has firmly established that sexual abuse impacts children's functioning in a variety of ways, but most especially in altering the brain's chemistry, causing behavioral and emotional dysregulation, challenging secure attachment, causing dissociation and other trauma-related problems and affecting a sense of self-worth and personal control and mastery. As a result, a combination of therapy approaches might be necessary since no one single model helps all children, and the sequence of treatment delivery is a relevant factor to success. In addition, even though there is a consensus about what treatment target areas should be addressed in therapy, there is no such agreement about what type of treatment is best for all abused children. Theraplay is an attachment-based, dyadic therapy that has great potential as an adjunctive therapy with sexually abused children and contributes greatly to treatment success.

Questions for reflection and continued learning

1. What are three reasons why it would be beneficial to focus primarily on building/re-establishing a safe and healthy attachment between a child and caregiver after the family has been impacted by child sexual abuse?

2. What is the importance of using safe and healthy touch when treating child sexual abuse, and how would you clarify your intentions and boundaries in a session with a child?

3. What are the considerations and justifications for using Theraplay integrated with another trauma-focused model to address the therapeutic goals for a child who has experienced sexual abuse? What factors would lead you to use Theraplay as the initial treatment or after a different model is used?

References

Arvidson, J., Kinniburgh, K., Howard, K., Spinazzola, J. *et al.* (2011). "Treatment of complex trauma in young children: Developmental and cultural consideration in application of the ARC intervention model." *Journal of Child and Adolescent Trauma, 4,* 34–51.

Blaustein, M. & Kinniburgh, K. (2018). *Treating Traumatic Stress in Children and Adolescents: How to Foster Resilience Through Attachment, Self-Regulation, and Competency* (second edition). New York, NY: Guilford Press.

Felitti, V., Anda, R., Nordenberg, D., Williamson, D.F. *et al.* (2019). "Relationship of childhood abuse and household dysfunction to many of the leading causes of death in adults: The adverse childhood experiences (ACE) study." *American Journal of Preventative Medicine, 56*(6), 774–786.

Finkelhor, D. (2009). "The prevention of childhood sexual abuse." *The Future of Children, 19*(2), 169–194.

Finkelhor, D., Shattuck, M.A., Turner, H.A. & Hamby, S.L. (2014). "The lifetime prevalence of child sexual abuse and sexual assault assessed in late adolescence." *Journal of Child and Adolescent Health, 55*, 329–333.

Gaskill, R. & Perry, B. (2013). "The Neurobiological Power of Play: Using the Neurosequential Model of Therapeutics to Guide Play in the Healing Process." In C. Malchiodi & D.A. Crenshaw (eds) *Play and Creative Arts Therapy for Attachment Problems* (pp.178–194). New York, NY: Guilford Press.

Gil, E. (2006). *Helping Abused and Traumatized Children: Integrating Directive and Nondirective Approaches.* New York, NY: Guilford Press.

Gil, E. (2012). "Trauma-Focused Integrated Play Therapy (TF-IPT)." In P. Goodyear-Brown (ed.) *Handbook of Child Sexual Abuse: Identification, Assessment, and Treatment* (pp.251–278). Hoboken, NJ: John Wiley & Sons.

Gil, E. (2017). *Post-Traumatic Play in Children: What Clinicians Should Know.* New York, NY: Guilford Press.

Hodges, M., Godbout, N., Briere, J., Lanktree, C. *et al.* (2013). "Cumulative trauma and symptom complexity in children: A path analysis." *Child Abuse and Neglect, 37*(11), 891–898.

Karakurt, G. & Silver, K.E. (2014). "Therapy for childhood sexual abuse survivors using attachment and family systems theory orientations." *American Journal of Family Therapy, 42*(1), 79–91.

Kezelman, C. & Stavropoulos, P. (2012). *The Last Frontier: Practice Guidelines for Treatment of Complex Trauma and Trauma Informed Care and Service Delivery.* Sydney: Advocates for Survivors of Sexual Abuse.

Lohrasbe, R. & Ogden, P. (2017). "Somatic resources: Sensorimotor psychotherapy approach to stabilizing arousal in child and family treatment." *Australian & New Zealand Journal of Family Therapy, 38*, 573–581.

National Child Traumatic Stress Network. (2019). *Sexual Abuse.* Retrieved from www.nctsn.org/what-is-child-trauma/trauma-types/sexual-abuse.

Perry, B.D. (2006). "Applying Principles of Neurodevelopment to Clinical Work with Maltreated and Traumatized Children." In N.B. Webb (ed.) *Working with Traumatized Youth in Child Welfare* (pp.27–52). New York, NY: Guilford Press.

Porges, S. (2011). *The Polyvagal Theory: Neurophysiological Foundations of Emotions, Attachment, Communication and Self-Regulation.* New York, NY: W.W. Norton and Company.

Ports, K., Ford, D. & Merrick, M. (2016). "Adverse childhood experiences and sexual victimization in adulthood." *Child Abuse and Neglect, 51*, 313–322.

Powell, B., Cooper, G., Hoffman, K. & Marvin, B. (2016). *The Circle of Security Intervention: Enhancing Attachment in Early Parent-Child Relationships.* New York, NY: Guilford Press.

Rubin, P.B., Lender, D. & Mroz-Miller, J. (2010). "Theraplay for Children with Histories of Complex Trauma." In P. Booth (ed.) *Theraplay: Helping Parents and Children Build Better Relationships Through Attachment-Based Play* (pp.359–404). San Francisco, CA: Jossey-Bass.

Sheinberg, M. & Fraenkel, P. (2001). *The Relational Trauma of Incest: A Family Based Approach to Treatment.* New York, NY: Guilford Press.

Silberg, J. (2013). *The Child Survivor: Healing Developmental Trauma & Dissociation.* New York, NY: Routledge.

van der Kolk, B.A. (2015). *The Body Keeps the Score: Brain, Mind, and Body in the Healing of Trauma.* London, UK: Penguin Books.

Wilcox, D., Richards, F. & O'Keefe, Z. (2004). "Resilience and risk factors associated with experiencing childhood sexual abuse." *Child Abuse Review, 13*(5), 338–352.

Chapter 9

Using Theraplay to Help Children who are Moving Families

Vivien Norris

Introduction

It is hard to imagine what a child goes through when they have to move family, sometimes multiple times. Even the concept of having to go through this experience feels alien. When faced with uncertainty and fear, a child will turn towards their known attachment figures for security and comfort. So what happens if the attachment figure is not coming and the child moves alone? How can they orient themselves, seek comfort and make some sense of what is happening to them? This chapter will explore what we, as professionals, might do to help children and the families involved in providing their care in this painful position.

Key points

1. All children who are fostered and adopted will face the profoundly difficult experience of moving family, sometimes multiple times. Moving family entails the loss of almost everything that is familiar to a child, and most crucially the loss of the child's main attachment figure. It is essential that the adults supporting this process find ways to mediate the child's inevitable distress as far as this is possible.

2. Fostered and adopted children have typically experienced developmental trauma (chronic relational trauma while in the care of their

primary carer) in their early months and years. This leaves them vulnerable to a range of difficulties (van der Kolk, 2015).

3. Theraplay as an intervention provides a very helpful framework for supporting children across family transitions (Norris, 2015). It can help carers get to know the child more deeply, facilitate emotional connection and provide a sequence of simple play interactions that can be used across the different family contexts, thereby creating a sense of continuity for the child. Theraplay also can provide regulatory support and a safe structure within which difficult conversations can take place.

4. Adaptations to Theraplay are made when it is used across family transition. Interventions begin within the fostering setting, continue through the introduction period and then into the adoption setting after the move. This means that two different sets of carers are involved, sometimes at the same time. The intervention starts with a dyadic focus (foster carer and child), moves to a group focus when the adopters are introduced (where both sets of carers are involved) and returns to a dyadic focus after the child has moved family (adopter and child). The main goal is to provide connection and continuity of experience across contexts, helping the child to feel safer and more understood.

5. Utilizing Theraplay across transitions has now been adapted for use in different family contexts and a clear model has been developed, called *By Your Side* (Norris, 2019). The principles of this approach are that all adults share an attachment and trauma-informed approach and are involved and supported. The emphasis throughout is on keeping the child's main attachment figure close by and supporting the child to seek comfort from them. Direct work sessions are provided across the whole process to give consistency and connection (using Theraplay) and to help create understanding and meaning for the child (integrating dyadic developmental psychotherapy (DDP) into the Theraplay) (Hughes, Golding & Hudson, 2019). Note: Countries differ in the way long-term care for children is provided. The work described in this chapter focuses on the transition from foster care to adoption in the UK but can be applied to other family contexts and countries.

Using an attachment and trauma-informed model for family transition support

Moving family is extremely stressful for any child. There are additional challenges for children who have had very difficult early years' experiences. Depending on the child's experience, the response to these stresses can play out in various ways. See Table 9.1 below.

Children who are moving family from foster care to adoption will typically have experienced developmental trauma in their early years, and so when we think about how best to support them over the transition to a new family, these vulnerabilities need to be taken into account. Where a parent is not able to provide sensitive care to their baby and child, for whatever reason, the child will find strategies to manage the best they can. They may become self-reliant and hide their needs or they may become highly distressed. The situation is extremely stressful for the baby or child. They are not mature enough to manage on their own and are frightened by what is happening around them. The combination of the lack of predictable and sensitive parental care alongside frightening or neglectful experiences (such as domestic violence, abuse and neglect) impacts the developing child in wide-ranging and profound ways. The term "developmental trauma" (van der Kolk, 2015) has been used to describe the range of impacts on a child. These include the child's response to stress, their ability to communicate thoughts and feelings and the development of control over their bodies, emotions and behaviors (physiological, emotional and behavioral regulation). Crucially the child's attachment relationships will be compromised and they may not experience a stable "felt sense of safety" or seek comfort when distressed (Porges, 2011).

The child is likely to have a fragile sense of trust in adults and a sensitivity to being triggered into a survival state of being, or to go back to earlier ways of relating when stressed. This means that although the child may have made progress in foster care, when they are under stress again (for instance, because they have to change family) they show earlier behaviors and may move away from rather than towards their main attachment figure. They are also likely to hide their fear and to give signals that they are fine and self-sufficient when they are feeling frightened (miscueing). In addition, their capacity to think and make sense of what is happening to them is likely to be highly compromised and exacerbated by fear. They may not be able to process and retain information or respond to logic, and their sense of time may be distorted. Foster carers will often report that things have been explained clearly to a child but *"they act as if they haven't heard it."* Alongside age-related development and a child's concept of time, children who are highly anxious may be able only to think in minutes or seconds, and any discussion of the future beyond that may be meaningless (Perry, 2009).

This obviously presents challenges in terms of how to be of most help to children who are moving family. We need to find ways to communicate important information to the child and help them express their experience (so that they have a sense of the narrative or story about what is happening to them) while helping them to make best use of their safe adults for support. Theraplay provides an ideal framework within which this support can be provided. The structured non-verbal sensory approach is accessible even to very young children, the attachment figure is centrally involved throughout, the relationship-focused activities can form a powerful sequence and ritual of connected play, and the overall structure provides predictability and safety within which difficult conversations can take place.

The *By Your Side* model (Norris, 2019) has been developed to keep the many needs of the child in mind and to try and support children to make use of their main attachment figure through the process. The model uses Theraplay sessions as the main framework and may also integrate some talking (DDP-based) during the quiet part of the session. The goal is to provide the child with an experience that someone is by their side through this most difficult of processes and that they do not have to manage alone. I will use the principles of the *By Your Side* model to illustrate the work in practice:

- Adults share an attachment and trauma-informed approach.

- Practitioner stays by the adults' side.

- Adults stay by the child's side.

- An attachment figure is always close by.

- The practitioner leads direct work.

- Consistency and connection are provided (Theraplay).

- A meaningful/coherent narrative is created (DDP).

Table 9.1: Transition process overview (Norris, 2019)

ISSUES →	IMPLICATIONS →	GOALS
• Fragile sense of safety and reliance on adults. • Child easily triggered into survival state (fight, flight, freeze) and into earlier ways of relating when stressed (self-sufficiency, presenting as if "fine," dysregulating). • Miscueing, hiding fear, trying to fit in and please adults. • Compromised sense of time and ability to process information (also age-related development). • Uncertainty likely to be filled by the child's fantasy and anxiety. • Fragmented sense of history, and sense that no one holds all the pieces—easier to block off difficult issues than to integrate. • Ending contact with birth family members—confusion, grief. • Attachments to adult figure come before new sibling attachments. If more than one child is moving, current sibling bond may undermine formation of reliance on new parent. • All of the above increases with length of exposure to trauma and number of moves.	• Promote development of attachment and reliance on adults even in short-term placements. • Close observation of what excites, regulates, calms. • Focus on child's felt sense of safety—assume fear underlies many behaviors. • Introduce attachment-forming interventions early. • Introduce idea of new parents only once they are ready to meet the child. • Repeat information simply, with visual cues. • Provide non-verbal sensory continuity across contexts. • Use child's history as "dictionary" to help understand behavior. Detailed and personalized—how the child shows stress, seeks comfort, specific details of events and people. • Hold joint sessions to provide connecting experiences as well as exploring difficult themes with main attachment figure alongside. Start while in foster placement and continue across introduction and after family move. • Ensure adult time for discussion—essential to increase the capacity of adults to bear inevitable distress and mediate the process on behalf of the child. • Mark the passage of time via non-verbal rituals. • Ensure that timings follow the needs of the child rather than being rigid and adult led.	Encourage child to form a strong attachment to their permanent family: • Adult able to interpret the child's cues accurately (such as being aware of miscueing) and respond to unmet need underneath the behavior. • New family able to understand, withstand and grow through challenges—to "keep going." • Adult can draw on understanding of the impact of the child's early experiences to make sense of behavior and remain empathetic, accepting, curious and playful. • Adult expects and makes sense of rejections and personal attacks within developmental trauma context. • Shared moments of connection and belonging. • Adult quickly initiates repair of relationship after ruptures in attunement. • Adult increasingly able to support the child's capacity to regulate via co-regulation. • Child turns to the adult for comfort when distressed. • Child takes the risk of sharing fear and confusion.

The role of the practitioner involved in facilitating this kind of work is to provide support to the adults as well as to provide a sequence of direct work sessions involving the child with their main attachment figures (i.e., initially the foster carer, then both foster carer and new parent, then new parent). The typical pattern of sessions using this model is given in Table 9.2 below.

Table 9.2: Typical sequence of sessions

Adult-only meetings to bring information together, review and plan at different points (a range of professionals could be involved).
MIM undertaken with the foster carers, if possible.
Four direct work sessions with foster carer and child prior to introductions.
Two direct work sessions during introductions (one of which involves foster carers and adopters together).
One adult review meeting mid-way through introductions.
Four to six direct work sessions with adopter and child after child has moved.
Telephone support as needed.

The sequence is adapted according to the particular needs of the family. In the following case study, I describe the process of facilitating a transition using Theraplay involving a sibling group of two children. In order to focus on some of the details, I describe more of the work with the older child.

CASE ILLUSTRATION

Connor (aged five) and Seren (aged three) were in short-term foster care with Nisha and Pete. They had already been through a lot in their short lives. They had experienced neglect, a lot of family chaos, multiple house moves and changes in carer (from birth mother, to grandmother, to auntie, to foster care), and had witnessed domestic abuse and experienced neglect while within their birth family. Since being taken into the care system they had lived in four different foster placements. The first placement was an emergency one as the children came into care unexpectedly, having been found outside unsupervised. They quickly moved into another placement but the carers found the level of crying and chaos created by the two children overwhelming and the children were moved again in an emergency. After a brief period in a third foster placement, Connor and Seren were living with Nisha and Pete, experienced carers who were providing an organized and caring atmosphere for the children. The children had been living with Pete and Nisha for a year, now and though Connor and Seren were not easy to care for, things had gradually improved. The decision was made (via the court process) that the children would be placed together in an adoptive family. Prospective adopters were being identified and the children had had their final contacts with their birth family. I was asked to facilitate some transition work to help the children make this move successfully.

There were many issues to address and I used the framework of the *By Your Side* model to help structure the work.

Principle 1: Adults share an attachment and trauma-informed approach

The aim is for the adults to share an overarching framework and approach to the transition. The adults come together to share what they know about the children, from the children's early years history and the foster carers' experience of parenting them. We are trying to develop a deeper understanding about what life has been like for them, what might lie underneath some of their behaviors and in particular what the foster carers' lived experience of parenting the children has been like. What is it like to be with them, to parent them, what might their behaviors mean and how might this impact the development of new relationships? This formulation process is often best achieved by organizing a meeting that involves all of the key adults. The meeting has a different emphasis from a typical planning or task-focused meeting and can be helpfully supported by training so that everyone involved has a good understanding of the impacts of developmental trauma on attachment and wider functioning.

 We discussed the children at an adults meeting. When I was asked to be involved, I started with a MIM with Pete and Nisha and so we had a detailed understanding of the specific patterns of each child. It was very helpful undertaking this MIM as it also allowed me to develop a relationship with Pete and Nisha and gain a sense of how well they knew the children, their parenting styles and the quality of the children's relationships with them. All of this information would be very useful in making sense of their responses as we moved towards the change in family.

In the adults meeting, Nisha and Pete described some different areas of concern around the care of the children. Whenever one of them was upset, both joined in with crying and drama (they appeared to be quite undifferentiated in their emotional responses), their behaviors escalated and Nisha and Pete had to separate them in order to be able to provide the soothing adult presence that the children needed to calm. Seren (the younger child) was enthusiastic and creative; she was able to play and form relationships, though she tended to be very indiscriminate, moving effortlessly between adults and seeking to have her needs met by whomever happened to be available (whether known or unknown to her). Connor, in contrast, was reticent and anxious and would try to be self-sufficient and manage things himself, and he found the nurturing part of being cared for really difficult. Through the discussion we formed a picture of two children with complex and different needs but were left with a sense of Connor being particularly vulnerable. He tended to move away from adult support, especially when stressed, and we anticipated (from Nisha and Pete's experience) that it could be harder for new parents to connect with him than with Seren.

We had obvious concerns about both children and I had some reservations about a joint placement, but this decision had been made. Although there was likely to be the need for some specialist therapeutic work with the children at a later stage, the task we faced was how to support all involved over the impending move. During this initial stage we were trying to forge strong adult relationships, develop a shared attachment and trauma-informed understanding of the children's issues, and agree on our approach.

Principle 2: Practitioner stays by the adults' side

When you are in a position of undertaking a piece of work which includes a range of adults with different roles, the likelihood of complex dynamics is high. This is made much more likely when the context is distressing. The process of moving a child from one family to another can easily become emotionally overwhelming for adults due to the varied perspectives and intensity of emotion. If we, the adults, are to really make sense of the child's experience we need to be able to bear facing their early years experience, the reason why they cannot stay with their birth family and the enormity of what it is we are doing. This requires really engaging with what it might be like to be a child in this situation.

Maintaining a position of openness and compassion can be hard. In many situations involving distress, we become self-protective and try to reassure or talk things up. This commonly happens across transition processes, with a positive picture of hope and excitement being presented and a lot of energy being put into concrete planning as a way to manage. This self-protective process has been usefully described as a "defence against anxiety" (Menzies-Lyth, 1988) and is manifest in the way in which adoption stories usually focus on excitement and hope rather than engaging with the mixed emotions, anxiety and fear the child may be carrying (Boswell & Cudmore, 2014).

What all of this means is that it is not enough just to focus on the direct work with the child. Someone needs to provide emotional containment for the adults, to help them make sense of what they are experiencing and to provide a sense of direction. Within the *By Your Side* model, this role is taken on by the practitioner delivering the direct Theraplay work (but it equally could be taken on by someone else in the system). The adults involved will need a high level of support so that they do not get caught up in unhelpful dynamics. This includes the various professionals as well as the prospective adopters. It is very helpful to keep asking: Where is the child in all of this? Why is it so hard for us to hold their experience at the front of our minds? With any piece of clinical work, and transition work in particular, there is a crucial role for the practitioner involved in containing and making sense of these adult dynamics.

 During the work with Conor and Seren, differences of opinion quickly emerged between the social worker representing the foster carers and the worker representing the adopters. They disagreed about the timing of the introductions, the adoption social worker arguing that Connor should move a week before Seren to allow time for him to develop a relationship with his new parents first (a sequential plan of introductions for siblings where the oldest child moves in first). In addition, the children's social worker felt a short introduction period would be best to save distressing the children too much. The discussions took on a combative atmosphere and were focused on planning. All perspectives came from good motivation, but the children's actual experiences were rarely in focus and so this became my initial task. I had to take great care not to join in with gossip or take sides, but rather to help each individual to feel heard and to try and help them to reorient their gaze onto what was actually happening for the children.

It was important to recognize that some "typical practice" for transitions appeared to be based on the short timeframes used for transitioning babies and there was less certainty about how to adjust this for older children. Drawing on the theoretical framework that underpins *By Your Side* was very helpful to keep me on track, and I used video clips from the MIM and initial Theraplay sessions to "bring the children into the room" during our discussions. The initial meeting with the adults that I had facilitated at the start became a useful reference point. This adult work continued throughout the transition period, with a high level of liaison, and on a couple of occasions I organized additional meetings with different adults. Through using acceptance, empathy and curiosity in my approach with the adults (drawing on the DDP model), they were more able to appreciate and stay with the children's experience.

Principle 3: Adults stay by the child's side

When the first two principles are adhered to it becomes easier to focus on the child's experience and to understand more clearly what kinds of support may help them. The child's core issues will come up within the MIM and Theraplay sessions and you can help the adult network interpret the child's responses from a developmental trauma and relationship perspective. The level of experience and training of the practitioner involved is obviously key.

 We decided to start with a Theraplay session involving both children and the foster carer. I facilitated a session that followed a typical sequence: entrance, check in (measuring and hello song), sequence of activities (bean-bag drop, bubble pop, a couple of circle songs, blanket run), then a couple of nurture activities involving a food snack and singing the personalized Twinkle song, before ending with a structured exit. Only Nisha was available, so the session involved me, Nisha and the two children. We did some activities in pairs, and others as a whole group, going in a circle one way and then the other. Some clear themes emerged. As anticipated, Seren was much more relaxed than Connor. She needed quite a high level of structure and scooping onto laps to keep her steady, but she was very able to engage in reciprocal and delightful interactions. Nisha was confident with her and they were enjoying each other. Connor, in contrast, was highly anxious and hypervigilant. He stared at me in an anxious way as if trying to work out what I wanted from him, and although he went along with what we were doing, had good eye contact and smiled, there was little sense of connection and we saw very few moments of genuine relaxed play.

Nisha and I continued our thinking about both children in the context of their history. Their styles of relating were very different. Nisha described Connor as being "cute looking" but as if "he wasn't really there." He would try to entertain adults and was very attentive to the impact he was having on others. Although he didn't seem that hard to care for (because he was compliant), Nisha described finding him really hard to feel close to. She felt she was providing practical parenting without a feeling of connection and this had troubled her all the way through his time with her. Because he seemed "okay," however, and no one else had seemed particularly worried, she had accepted that this was how he was. As we talked more, her feelings of guilt about "not liking him much" came to the fore. I could see how this might come about from my brief experience of trying to connect with Connor.

Connor was compliant and smiled but this felt like miscueing. His interactions were emotionally flat and tense. As Nisha described this consistent pattern over the past year, I started to feel concerned about the new adopters and the risk of blocked care if things continued as they were. Blocked care describes an emotional state that parents can experience when they are parenting children who do not have trust and are hard to connect with. Over time, the parent becomes emotionally exhausted and their previous capacity for warmth and responsive care diminishes (Baylin & Hughes, 2016). It was interesting that Nisha's level of discomfort had not really come across in either the profile she had written about Connor, nor in the initial adults meeting. I felt this most likely related to her own sense of shame about her feelings as well as wanting to promote a positive picture and create hope for the future. I talked frankly with Nisha about the concept of blocked care and she agreed that she was experiencing this with respect to Connor, though not towards Seren. Nisha had heard of the concept but had not explored it in any depth and had not realized that it was possible to have such different feelings about two siblings. It also appeared that the short-term nature of the foster placement had meant that Nisha could "let some things go" in the hope that time would help.

Obviously, it would have been helpful for this family to have had Theraplay support earlier in the placement and I would be recommending some intervention for the future, but for now we were preparing for a change in the family. I needed to be pragmatic and work out what could be helpful in this context. The MIM and this first session had already proved very useful. We were gaining a deeper understanding of the issues, and specifically the difficulties Connor was facing regarding connecting with close carers. We thought about his early years experience and hypothesized that his exposure to high levels of unpredictable violence in the household and the lack of sensitive and reciprocal care he had received from the adults had left him frightened, vigilant and trying to manage on his own. He did not have a sufficient felt sense of safety to engage and did not really know how to be in a reciprocal relationship. In many ways, the work with Connor would be akin to working with an infant, trying to find tiny ways to draw him into a genuinely reciprocal interaction.

There were issues regarding Seren too; her level of indiscriminate behavior was a worry. After discussion, we decided that we would do one more session with the children together, so that both children could become more familiar with the Theraplay and also both be present when we first started conversations about moving family, and that after that we would have a separate session with Connor. Alongside this, we formed a mini-sequence of play activities (lasting a few minutes) which Nisha agreed to play each day at home with both children (we chose bean-bag drop, ring a roses and the Twinkle song).

Nisha also revisited the notes she had written for the new parents and added more detail about how she experienced relating with Connor. She focused on examples of how hard he found reciprocity (to and fro relating), the things that he seemed to find most manageable and the subtle ways she had provided some soothing support, because direct nurture was rejected.

Principle 4: An attachment figure is always close by

Although it is well established that children feel safest when close to a safe attachment figure to whom they can turn for comfort, it is surprising how often therapeutic work is undertaken, or important information shared, with children in isolation. An example of this might be when a social worker comes to talk to a child but the foster carer is not in the room.

The principle of having an attachment figure nearby applies to all elements of transition work, from conversations with social workers, to the inclusion of an attachment figure in therapy sessions. It impacts too on what happens when new parents are introduced into the family across the introductions period and what messages are given to the child.

Keeping an attachment figure close by is an integral part of the *By Your Side* approach. At each stage, the adults observe who the child turns to when stressed and do everything they can to "buffer" the child from stress via the support of this figure. In the early stages of any transition, the key attachment figure will be the foster carer, who has a critical role as the person who knows the child best. Over the introductions period, as the adoptive parent becomes more familiar, the situation shifts such that the child becomes more reliant on the new person. The process of forming a new attachment is gradual and the child faces the loss of one relationship alongside the gradual deepening of another. Even after the move, the child is likely to have strong feelings about the loss of their foster carer, and the process of mourning this loss and forming the new attachments takes time. It is obviously very helpful for everyone involved to receive training and guidance on this issue and to share an expectation that the foster carers will visit the child soon after the move and maintain in some way a relationship with the new family. This sounds straightforward in theory but can be emotionally hard and requires agreement and support.

Different elements of the *By Your Side* approach link to this theme: the bringing together of the key attachment figures to try and create an atmosphere of "working together as a team" on behalf of the child; keeping the main attachment figure involved throughout; the professionals and new parents actively deferring to the knowledge and experience of the primary attachment figure (e.g., the adopter defers to the foster carer in front of the child: "I'm not sure. What do you think, Nisha, you know what she likes best?"); and the provision of a joint Theraplay session (or more than one) during the introductions period.

I had made various attempts to keep Nisha and Pete central to the support around the children, beginning with the initial meeting, and since then had worked hard to promote a positive relationship between them and the new parents. Nisha expressed her appreciation that her role was being acknowledged and we could see her increase in confidence as we went through the transition process. Her previous experience of transitions had been to take a step back, to "give the new parents space," but she could see that there were times when the children were struggling and she hadn't stepped in. She confided, "I didn't want people to think I was over-involved or being disruptive."

Within this new shared approach Nisha felt that her role, as the person who knew the children best, was being valued and we could see multiple ways in which she helped the new parents to get to know the children well. She kept close by to monitor the children's well-being and adjusted the pace if they were finding things hard. I had also prepared the new adopters (Tony and David) and they came into the process with an understanding of what to expect and permission to ask for help from Nisha and Pete. This meant that they could only ask, in front of the children, when they weren't sure of something, and the message "we're just getting to know each other, I'm just going to check in with Nisha and Pete" helped the children to feel the ongoing presence of their safe figures.

One example of this came on day two of the introductions. The day before, when the children met their new dads for the first time, Connor had surprised everyone by flinging himself on them immediately and looking extremely at ease with them. On day two, he asked "new Daddy" (Tony) to come upstairs with him to his room. Nisha followed behind. As they got to the room, Connor went inside with Tony and then shut the door leaving Nisha outside the bedroom. This was an unexpected situation, but because of the preparation and shared understanding of the approach, the adults could work together to ensure that Nisha (Connor's safe adult figure) was brought back into the room. Tony said, "Hey, we need Nisha in here, she's helping me to get to know all the ways you need to be looked after," and he opened the door.

Another very concrete way of demonstrating to the child that the most important adults in their life are working together on their behalf is through the experience of a joint Theraplay session in which the overarching message is that the current attachment figures (the foster carers) are showing the new parents "all the special ways we play together." This kind of session requires sensitive and capable facilitation and good adult preparation as it can be emotionally intense. The session is set up more like a Group Theraplay session, with activities going around the circle in different directions. The most intense nurturing elements are not included at this time in order to keep the level of intensity manageable. If the adults involved can manage this kind of session, it communicates a very powerful message to the child.

 We were in the middle of the introductions period and were getting ready for our joint session, involving both the foster carers and adopters. In order to keep the number of adults down a bit we decided that only Nisha would be involved, along with the two new parents and me. In discussion with Nisha, we felt that she and I could manage the children between us. In another situation I might well have included a colleague to help (i.e., one of us to lead and the other to manage issues that cropped up). I had a preparation session with both foster carer and adopters and went through the planned session exactly as it would happen so they knew what to expect. I let them all know that for the children this joint session would be intense and that they might be confused about where to sit. Now that they were getting to know their new dads there might be a sense of Nisha's lap not feeling quite right. I reassured them that they could just follow my lead, that I would keep the session flowing. I talked with them about how it was natural that they would want to look intently at the children but to try not to stare too much. Everyone was open to trying the session but the adopters were understandably anxious. I organized the session so that we played a few of the familiar activities that the children had played in the previous sessions and integrated a song that was familiar to the children.

We all came in in a line holding hands and sat down in a circle, settled and I introduced the session saying it would be a bit different today because we would be showing the new dads "all the games we play." I started everyone off with the hello song which we sang with actions as a group: "Here I am, Here I am, How do you do?" We moved into passing a lotion blob around the group and then to checking whether the next person's nose was warm or cold and then whether their hair was soft or prickly. Seren, as anticipated, appeared quite relaxed and was a little restless but managed fine. Connor, who had been very over-familiar with his new parents since meeting them a week ago, became more hesitant. It was fascinating watching how the structure of the touch activity slowed him down and we saw him hold back before touching David's nose. I immediately took over, touched David's nose on Connor's behalf, so as not to put him under pressure, and we continued round the circle. The same thing happened the next time round and I touched David's hair for Connor, stating that it felt a bit prickly. This ritual felt important and very different from the way in which he had been flinging himself on both his new dads during the previous week (which had been concerning all of us). The session continued in a similar vein, with Connor showing a healthy hesitation. During the snack I decided to move him to Nisha so that he could relax a bit into her familiar body.

Principle 5: The practitioner leads direct work

This multi-session sequence of direct work, alongside the support of the carers, is provided by one skilled worker across the whole transition period. This worker becomes a bridge connecting the two contexts; the worker's specific role is to get alongside the key individuals and to keep the child's needs and experience central throughout. The direct work includes sessions within the foster care setting, sessions involving all during introductions, sessions with the adopters after the move, and various adults meetings. The content of the sessions themselves is based on the typical Theraplay protocol. Whether the session is facilitated as a dyadic session or a group session will depend on the number of people involved and the stage of the process. Ideally you will want to include several dyadic sessions involving individual children with their main carer. This is obviously straightforward with a one-child transition but takes more thought where you are supporting a sibling group. In this situation, it is usually most helpful to have a session involving all the children at first (i.e., a group session) and then to work with the most vulnerable child for a few dyadic sessions. The joint foster carer-adopter session during introductions is always more akin to a group session. There are variations in how the sessions are organized depending on the family. As can be seen in the case illustration, the decisions about exactly how many sessions to have, with whom and how to structure them can be highly individual to the situation. The overarching aim is to provide the child with a sense of safety and continuity. A further aim is to support the carer/adopters and enable them to develop confidence and feel supported, to feel that someone is "by their side" too.

Principle 6: Consistency and connection are provided (Theraplay)

A specific strength of Theraplay is the way in which non-verbal and sensory-based connection can be provided so that the children experience it as direct and genuine. When a child is facing the loss of almost everything familiar to them, the moments of connection with a safe adult figure both within and outside the session are deeply reassuring: "Maybe I'm not on my own after all."

When a child in a stable care setting receives Theraplay, the practitioner typically focuses on areas of difficulty and works gradually over a number of sessions to make progress in a purposeful way. However, over a transition period, so much is going on and the child is facing so many challenges that this is not the best time to focus on areas of difficulty. More importantly, the Theraplay work enables a closeness, a sense of connection and relationship safety at a time of high anxiety. For this reason, sessions will tend to focus on activities that go well (for parent and child) and steer away from more problematic areas. The aim is to develop a sequence of play that helps the child to remain regulated and feel connected to their main carer. Some of the most impactful activities have a strong symbolic message and include themes of going away from a carer and back (e.g., peek-a-boo, "you just can't see me but I'm still here" and running under a raised blanket back and forth between practitioner and parent, which is like a way of practicing going away from and back to a safe figure) and those that communicate togetherness (e.g., singing together and matching games).

 After the move, we had a session involving the whole family. Connor and Seren rushed up to greet me and were more friendly than usual. I began the session with an entrance and then singing together. Both children showed deep pleasure in the familiarity of the structure and Connor leant close to me as we sang. I repeated a series of activities that both children had played in the sessions involving their foster carers, and Tony and David ably supported the children. It was very noticeable that the over-familiar response that we had seen from Connor towards Tony had changed. Connor was, in fact, showing more interest in me and maneuvered himself onto my lap early on in the session, and as we did a bean-bag drop in a circle, he pushed Tony's hand away stating that he could do it by himself. I could see that both of these things might create anxiety for Tony and David. My interpretation of Connor's warmth towards me was that I had now (for a temporary period) become the safest lap, as Connor was now experiencing the reality of the new relationships. I had known Connor longer than Tony and David and had also known Nisha and Pete (whom Connor was missing terribly), so this draw towards me was understandable. During the session I allowed this closeness and tried to provide the family with a simple and familiar sequence of enjoyable activities. The purpose was as much to provide a link to the past as to be together in this new family grouping, and the safety of the Theraplay structure allowed us all to see how the children responded. I followed up with Tony and David by phone after the session to hear their reflections on the session and to talk with them about how the children were settling more broadly.

In the following session, just Connor and Tony attended and we were able to address more specific rejections that Connor was showing towards Tony. As before, in the bean-bag drop, Connor pushed Tony's hands to the side repeatedly. I intervened and said, "I know you can do this on your own but we like to help you," and I encouraged Tony to place his hands close to Connor's to catch the bean bag. In this small adjustment we were giving Connor an important message of support, whether or not he felt he wanted it in that moment. There were other similar examples during the session.

When I spoke with Tony after the session he mentioned many small ways in which Connor was trying to be self-sufficient, like not wanting Tony to help him do up his shoes for instance. Though it was difficult, Tony was able to reflect on these small "rejections" without taking them too personally. He showed that he had understood the importance of these signals from Connor and the work of the new relationship began in a thoughtful way.

Principle 7: A meaningful/coherent narrative is created (DDP)

One of the impacts of multiple changes of family experienced by children who enter the looked-after system is a fragmented sense of history. There is no longer one adult who holds the memories of events and incidents of the baby and young child's story. Events, special preferences and everyday rituals that may have been crucial to the child may become blurred and forgotten. When children are old enough to express their views verbally, a common theme of distress is about details which have been overlooked by the adults: "I didn't get to say goodbye to the dog," "I lost my teddy," "She doesn't know how I like my toast."

In any transition work it is essential to find ways to help the child to develop a sense of coherence about what has happened and is happening to them. This can be hard to achieve when the child is very young and stressed, but there are many ways to promote a coherent narrative. Examples include: the provision of detailed notes that the foster carer provides for the new parents; the adults finding ways to weave key information into daily conversations; the provision of repeated rituals and time markers; and processing via play and therapeutic stories. Discussing these approaches in any detail is outside the scope of this chapter, but the Theraplay framework of sessions provides an ideal context in which some difficult conversations can take place. Once the child is familiar with the session structure then a talking element to the work can be easily added around the snack. The approach that fits most easily with Theraplay is dyadic developmental psychotherapy (Hughes *et al.*, 2019). Below is a brief example of integrating DDP work into the Theraplay sessions.

 We had added some symbolic play into the sessions with Connor, first using mini-figures to tell a simple story of what had happened to him and then using puppets to play out some of the repeated scenarios in Connor's story. We spent about 10–15 minutes doing this after the snack. In one session, Connor took two baby owl puppets and made them do all manner of naughty and dangerous things while Tony and I (being parent characters) tried to save them. "Hey Daddy, those little owls need a bit of help, they're dangling upside down; oh my goodness, they're going to fall, quick! You'd better get over there ready to catch them." Tony gamely took on the part of being a rabbit trying to protect the little owls. Through this play we explored themes such as "If I'm naughty will you still keep me?" and "Is this new parent quick enough for me?" The message I gave in the narrative was that everyone was getting to know each other and it would take time to see. As Connor experienced that we were accepting of his mixed feelings about the idea of moving, he became bolder and more expressive and over the course of the sessions we developed a clear sense of the issues that were in his mind. We ended each session with a couple of Theraplay games so that the session maintained the familiar structure and there was a clear ending.

The work with Seren did not include this narrative element as we felt that providing the safety and connection of Theraplay was containing enough for her at this point. As the work came to a close, we wrote an individualized therapeutic story for each child (Norris, 2018).

Conclusion

The process of supporting children to move family is complex and it can be hard to know how best to help them make some sense of what is happening to them. The range of practice in the area of family transitions is highly divergent and has been little researched and yet the impact on the many thousands of children who have to move family is profound and can significantly affect their future relationships.

Our experience (now tried and tested in different situations) is that the use of Theraplay as an organizing framework can be very powerful across major transitions (including different kinds of family transitions and other transitions such as reintegration into school). The Theraplay element is often combined with some DDP-based narrative work, finding ways to help the child form a sense of their "story," and also includes a level of adult-focused support. Through the sensitive provision of Theraplay the child can be helped to feel some *sense of safety* and to *feel connected* with those adults in a genuinely reciprocal manner. Only with this relationship scaffolding in place are they able to begin to make some sense of their narrative.

The model also provides a framework which supports the foster carers in their transition and provides a platform for the new parents to develop their relationship with their child. As the adults are emotionally held, so this feeling is communicated to the child.

Questions for reflection and continued learning

1. Can you identify the adult issues that you would face in your role which might make it hard to keep the child's experience central?

2. What are some practical adjustments you could make to your practice to help children in transition feel heard?

3. How could your organization incorporate the key principles of the *By Your Side* model into their transitions framework?

References

Baylin, J. & Hughes, D.A. (2016). *The Neurobiology of Attachment-Focused Therapy: Enhancing Connection and Trust in the Treatment of Children and Adolescents.* New York, NY: W.W. Norton and Company.

Boswell, S. & Cudmore, L. (2014). "'The children were fine': Acknowledging complex feelings in the move from foster care to adoption." *Adoption and Fostering, 38*(1), 5–21.

Hughes, D., Golding, K. & Hudson, J. (2019*). Healing Relational Trauma with Attachment-Focused Interventions: Dyadic Developmental Psychotherapy with Children and Families.* New York, NY: W.W. Norton and Company.

Menzies-Lyth, I. (1988). *Containing Anxiety in Institutions: Selected Essays.* London, UK: Free Association Books.

Norris, V. (2015). "Not Again, Little Owl: Transitions from Foster Care to Adoption." In C. Archer, C. Drury & J. Hills (eds) *Healing the Hidden Hurts: Transforming Attachment and Trauma Theory into Effective Practice with Families, Children and Adults* (pp.88–101). London, UK: Jessica Kingsley Publishers.

Norris, V. (2018). *Not Again Little Owl.* London, UK: The Family Place.

Norris, V. (2019). *By Your Side: Practitioner Guide. Support for Children Moving Families.* London, UK: The Family Place.

Perry, B.D. (2009). "Examining child maltreatment through a neurodevelopmental lens: Clinical applications of the neurosequential model of therapeutics." *Journal of Loss and Trauma, 14,* 240–255.

Porges, S.W. (2011). *The Polyvagal Theory: Neurophysiological Foundations of Emotions, Attachment, Communication, and Self-Regulation.* New York, NY: W.W. Norton and Company.

van der Kolk, B. (2015). *The Body Keeps the Score: Mind, Brain and Body in the Transformation of Trauma.* New York, NY: Penguin Books.

Chapter 10

Theraplay with Families Affected by Domestic Violence

Donna M. Gates

Introduction

All around the world, families are exposed to domestic violence (DV), whether experiencing abuse themselves, witnessing it or knowing someone who has been affected. From physical to verbal abuse, the effects are complex and multi-dimensional, impacting both the child's and the caregiver's sense of self and their coping, relational and cognitive skills. Theraplay is an ideal model for working with a child and a non-offending caregiver because of the model's primary focus on establishing the relational safety that builds resilience. This chapter presents key issues affecting those who experience domestic violence, focuses on the effects of emotional abuse, which is the core element of all abuse, and offers resources for more study. It describes how Theraplay can help in the healing process by following five guidelines.

Key points

1. Work with the non-offending caregiver to establish stability before working with that caregiver and child.

2. Expect secret-keeping, as it is a protective mechanism within the family system.

3. View "taking charge" by "parentified" children as their shield against feeling powerless.

4. Use Theraplay's *structure* to provide an experience of safety in relationship and *nurture* to encourage a sense of self-worth.

5. Use Theraplay's *engagement, challenge* and play to provide the impetus for change.

Recommendation

I recommend dyadic Theraplay for a non-offending caregiver and child as a reparative therapy once they are no longer in the DV situation— that is, either the offender has been removed from the home or the non-offending caregiver has moved with the children into a safer environment for a sufficient time such that they are able to experience a basic sense of safety. Living in a vigilant survival mode will not allow for the regulatory capacity needed to focus on social-emotional needs! I also want to note that although I have used Theraplay within male abuser groups (Gates, 2010), this is beyond the scope of this chapter. The use of Theraplay with offenders is more complex and requires more treatment and preparation.

Terminology

There are several terms currently in use for relational violence and they often are used interchangeably: "interpersonal violence" (IPV) is a broad term that includes personal relationships beyond the family context; "family violence" and "domestic violence" specifically refer to violence within the family unit and the effects for the abused partner and for the children; "intimate partner violence" (also shortened to IPV) refers specifically to violence within the couple relationship, though the effects on the children are usually also noted (National Child Traumatic Stress Network, 2019). I will use "domestic violence" (DV), referring to that which happens within a family unit of any type, since it is prevalent in much of the literature about this subject and because my focus in this chapter will be the effects and treatment of violence within the family. I will use the term "partner" to refer to any intimate couple relationship, whether or not the couple is married and whether they are the same or different gender; and "caregiver" will refer to anyone who is in a parenting role within the family unit. In addition, while being abusive is not gender specific, this chapter will often refer to the non-offending caregiver as "she," since the risk of harm and death from violence is higher for women than for men (Meyer & Frost, 2019).

Effect of DV on the child

Children do not need to be directly abused themselves for DV to have traumatizing effects; witnessing abuse/violence within the child's constellation of relationships can have harmful effects. The effect on the child depends on several mitigating factors: the severity of the event, the proximity to the event, caregivers' reactions, prior history of trauma, family and community factors. Most significant is the presence of a safe, caring person who is able to provide some soothing reassurance to the child and to acknowledge the child's feelings and the reality that the violence is not okay. This person might be another family member or friend, a neighbor or a therapist. Since young children have fewer coping skills, are more dependent on the care of adult caregivers and have less life experience for comparison of "How bad is this?" they are likely to experience any situation of anger or loss as more significant than an adult might experience it. Too often, the adults within a family system deny or minimize the impact on the children, especially very young children, and in the earlier stages of family violence. However, children see and hear things that occur within a highly conflictual family context, and they experience a number of emotions, including confusion (What is happening and why?), fear and anxiety (What will happen now? Will someone get hurt? What should I do? Who will protect me/us?), shame/guilt (Am I to blame? Why couldn't I have stopped it?), anger (Why does this keep happening? Why won't he/she/they stop it?) and helplessness (I try but it keeps happening! I'm just a kid!). When unable to share and process these emotions, the child may become vigilant and overly responsible to assuage adults, charming and entertaining to distract them, quiet and hidden to avoid them, or they may act out the emotions in a variety of ways. For more information, see Lundy Bancroft's (2004) book *When Dad Hurts Mom*.

Emotional abuse as the core element of all abuse

Emotional abuse is rarely a single incident, but "usually involves a pattern of abusive events" (Dugan & Hock, 2006, p.4). This pattern includes not only words but also attitudes displayed in actions, gestures, stance, tones and facial expressions, which communicate to the recipient a lack of worth, a lack of safety and a lack of competence/capacities. Emotional abuse includes intimidation, direct or implied threats, demeaning names or "jokes," criticism and accusations of one's character/self/role, and interference in the other's decision making and life experiences or responsibilities. "Life in the family changes when a man's abusiveness enters the picture" (Bancroft, 2004, p.3), fostering tension in all the relationships in the family and creating a variety of responses. Even if the abuser behaves "nicely" for a time, the uncertainty of when it will end is always present, and often the child is confused by the abuser's description of situations: casting blame, never taking responsibility and often sounding very reasonable. This is the manipulation that weaves throughout emotional abuse and undermines trust not only of the other, but also of one's own feelings and thoughts. This manipulation has a "crazy-making" effect that teaches members of a family experiencing abuse: "don't feel/don't tell/don't trust." For more information, see Patricia Evans (2010) *The Verbally Abusive Relationship*.

Although emotional abuse persists throughout other types of abuse, its insidious and devastating effects often are hidden, so people outside the family who might counter the powerful messages conveyed to the victim remain unaware of the messages and their eroding impact. Because the perpetrator of abuse often behaves very differently to people who are outside of the immediate family relationships, victims fear not being believed if they reveal the abuse to others. Even when one has had a secure start in life, ongoing abuse can erode the positive base.

Typically, the abused caregiver as well as the child feels alone and unsupported, insecure, powerless and incapable, and certainly fearful. Will this get worse? Will it be better if I stay or if I leave? Where would I go even if I did leave? How could I provide for myself and my children? And so on. In addition, the caregiver typically feels full of shame from questioning their core sense of self, their life choices and their powerlessness to prevent the abuse, to protect themselves and their child, or to leave the abuser (Walker, 2017). Even another non-abusive family member who steps in to care for the child may experience all of these feelings except perhaps for the sense of shame.

Effective interventions for witnesses and recipients of abuse

Bruce Perry (2006) lists six core elements of experience for healing trauma: relational/safe; relevant/developmentally matched; repetitive/ patterned; rewarding/pleasurable; rhythmic/resonant with neural patterns; and respectful/taking the child, family and cultural values into account. Each of these elements is a part of the Theraplay approach. Let's look at the guidelines for use of the Theraplay model for treating a child-caregiver dyad affected by DV.

1. Work with the non-offending caregiver before beginning sessions with the child

The first essential aspect of therapy for children who have experienced DV is to work with the non-offending caregiver in order to establish the stability and safety necessary for working on the relational goals of Theraplay. The non-offending caregiver will have been affected by the same "crazy-making" systemic patterns as the child. The importance of this work with the caregiver is supported by Bancroft as he identifies key elements for children from family violence to heal. While naming such elements as safety, connection to others (family, friends, self), ability to express feelings and be heard and opportunities to release distressing feelings, he firmly states, "The single most important avenue for your children's recovery is their relationship with you [the mom/non-abusing caregiver]" (2004, p.268).

So what does the non-offending caregiver need? First, to *gain information* about:

- the patterns of DV, especially regarding the core emotional abuse

- the personal rights which all humans need to have respected, but which are violated in DV

- how an abuser perceives personal interactions and why the victim's attempts to promote understanding have not worked

- what intervention the abuser would need for things to change

- precautions and preparations for remaining in the home with the abuser or for potentially leaving. (Bancroft, 2004; Dugan & Hock, 2006; Evans, 2010; National Center on Domestic and Sexual Violence, 2016)

This information can begin to help alleviate the shame that is the inheritance of abuse. The second need of the non-abusing caregiver is empathy for their difficulty in considering and enacting changes, given the destabilizing effects of the DV patterns they have experienced. The third need may be their own treatment for any mental health issues resulting from their experience of DV.

If the caregiver is still living in the home with the abuser, it is important to begin talking about the inner and relational tension that can arise when one is learning a new way to relate while returning home to the abusive system. This may become a new incentive for a caregiver to work with the practitioner and other support people to effect change. However, a safety plan always needs to be discussed and reviewed so that the new experiences do not lead the caregiver to inadvertently put herself and the child at more risk through new confrontations with the abuser. This sharing of information and discussion of safe decision making and safety planning requires additional caregiver sessions, either before or in parallel with the Theraplay, as this processing and reflection take time.

Although the amount of work needed to help a caregiver understand the dynamics of DV and the long-term effects for self and the child and that the available resources and options for change may vary from one caregiver to another, this preparation is the prerequisite for building the caregiver's self-efficacy, emotional availability and ability to protect and connect with the child. Addressing the three needs above (absorbing new information, receiving empathy for the difficulty in making changes, and receiving any needed individual treatment) will be the foundation for Theraplay's relational work to make progress and hope for sustaining gains.

2. Recognize secret-keeping as a protective mechanism

Both the child and the non-offending caregiver affected by DV have often learned "don't tell" as a way to protect themselves from incurring more abuse, from experiencing increased shame and from the fear of losing the caregiver, even though abusive. A non-offending caregiver may stay with the abuser to protect herself/her child or because she has been demeaned or isolated until she does not feel confident of having the skills, capacities or resources to provide adequately for herself and the children apart from the abuser. The fear may cause a child who has experienced domestic violence to be clingy, have separation anxiety when apart from caregivers and siblings, and even state desires to be with the abuser. These may also be the thoughts for children whose fear leads to aggressive behavior, impulsive or reckless behavior, an inability to concentrate, or emotional numbing. The thought is "What will happen if I am not there to stop the fight/to distract the abuser/to call for help/to protect the victims of the attack?" Consequently, no one tells things that could lead to awareness of the abuse, because "it could trigger the abuser and things could get worse." Even when children find a safe haven, they may avoid attaching due to misguided loyalties to the others in the family and fears of possible repercussions. Sometimes it is difficult to determine the nature of any suspected abuse; but since the effects are frequently the same whether the abuse is physical or emotional in nature or whether the abuse was witnessed or directly experienced by the child, the potential persists for Theraplay to be an effective intervention to lead to revealing and healing.

In several family cases, no evidence of domestic violence is revealed in the gathering of the family history, the patterns seen in the MIM, or the early caregiver sessions. In other cases, the offending parent had been through treatment for anger management and substance abuse and both parents profess that no abuse is continuing. Both the children and the caregivers can seem sufficiently stable and the living situations sufficiently safe, so I move carefully, slowly and thoughtfully into the dyadic Theraplay, with one caregiver and one child at each session. Although there is no one defining signal, I often sense a tension in the child between accepting the interactions with me and then becoming aggressive or avoidant with the caregiver, or enjoying the interactions until time to go home but then suddenly becoming physically dysregulated. Since there may be other reasons also for these reactions, I take note of this and proceed with careful planning and increased attunement, usually inserting a caregiver session next to explore and wonder about what might be triggering these reactions in the child. After a few dyadic sessions and one or two caregiver sessions, I frequently find that participation in the Theraplay model leads to either a caregiver or a child revealing some of their hidden fears or hurts. The gentle, kind relational interactions seem to create an environment of trust and goodwill more quickly than my other family therapy techniques, and empower someone within the system to break the secrecy in some small way that leads me back to the importance of further work with the caregiver to promote true safety building.

As the caregiver in treatment becomes able to talk about the abuse and to be more supportive and present with her child, the practitioner can guide her in ways to talk about this with the child and to help the child learn when and with whom to speak up about any needs, worries and questions the child may have. At the end of this chapter ("A final note about Theraplay for families who have experienced DV"), I give an example about listening and responding to a child's expressed experience of an abusive parent.

3. Create moments of empowerment to overcome a sense of powerlessness

Children who have experienced DV, especially an only child or the eldest child, typically experience the paradox of "parentification" while feeling powerless. In witnessing abuse between the caregivers, the child feels the burden to protect the caregiver victim and/or younger siblings by intervening somehow to stop the violence. Simultaneously, the child feels the weakness that comes from fear and from lack of life experience and accumulated coping skills. If children do successfully intervene in the aggression, they end up in an emotional double-bind—feeling more responsibility to intervene, while experiencing additional aloneness in the consequent stress, additional vigilance and possibly greater fear of reprisal. Even the non-offending caregiver frequently does not praise the child's efforts to protect fellow family members from abuse; that caregiver may see the intervention as dangerous for the child and/or as "making things worse" by escalating the unpredictable nature of the abusing caregiver.

The non-offending caregiver frequently experiences this same sense of paralyzed responsibility. Consequently, this caregiver either may react aggressively towards the offender or towards the children in order to feel less helpless, or may just comply so as to mollify the offender and move past the moment of helplessness. Although neither aggression nor compliance works effectively to address the sense of helplessness, these learned responses mean that both child and caregiver may have difficulty on the one hand trusting and following another leader and on the other hand risking trying something new.

Thus, we need to work to empower both child and caregiver if we are to help them trust and follow as we guide them to try new things. A child feels empowered when:

- someone notices her strengths and praises her efforts rather than achievements
- he feels his own self-efficacy in interactions
- she sees her non-offending caregiver taking steps towards change and becoming more present.

For a caregiver, it is empowering to:

- learn about the dynamics of DV and available resources for help
- be supported in slow-paced change
- have their feelings and motivations validated
- receive affirmation for the positive things they do.

4. Use Theraplay structure and nurture to create safety and self-worth

Theraplay can provide, for both child and non-offending caregiver, new messages which can regulate, soothe and eventually empower the dyad. These messages bring hope of something very different from the DV experience of anxious uncertainty, aloneness and unworthiness. Using the chart *How the Dimensions of Theraplay Meet the Needs of Children and Caregivers* created at The Theraplay Institute (Lindaman, 2015), we will reflect on the impact of these significant messages within each of Theraplay's four dimensions and within the context of play.

Table 10.1: Structure

The message of structure for the child	The message of structure for the caregiver
Adults behave in organized, predictable and kind ways.	Even if you could not protect the child in the past, you can do so now.
Your caregiver can be trustworthy and keep you safe. Your caregiver can help you when you are distressed or uncomfortable. You don't have to take care of yourself.	You can help the child calm down. You can set up routines in play and daily life that will reassure the child. You can set limits and guide behavior without being punitive. When you help your child manage their emotional ups and downs, they eventually learn self-control.

The *structure* which the Theraplay practitioner provides creates a new template for what an adult can be like: a model that contrasts with the messages learned by a child affected by DV. Within a DV family system, the child may see two simplified role models: an abusive caregiver who is unpredictable and scary, and a non-abusive caregiver who is unable to protect him. The Theraplay practitioner can provide a third model: an adult who is predictable and can be trusted to keep him safe and supported, so he does not have to take care of everything himself. Likewise, the caregiver messages begin to reassure and empower the caregiver that someone sees her as capable of learning to protect, calm and help her child. These new constructs are built over time, through repeated interactions between the practitioner and the caregiver as well as between the practitioner and the dyad, slowly shaping a new inner working model for each about self and other: life can become less chaotic, more manageable, more cooperative and more peaceful, even though not perfect.

In order to receive this new model that caregivers can be helpful, the child must experience a sense of self-worth. Activities in the nurture dimension help convey these messages.

Table 10.2: Nurture

The message of nurture for the child	The message of nurture for the caregiver
Your caregiver can help you feel better. Your caregiver can figure out and provide what you need.	You can learn how to read your child's cues. You can meet your child's needs.
Even if touch and physical closeness were frightening in the past, they can feel safe and good. Your caregiver can calm and soothe you.	You can figure out the best way to calm and soothe your child. Caring for a child isn't spoiling him or rewarding his bad behavior. Gentle touch is an important way to connect with and soothe a child.

Through the structured and nurturing interactions the practitioner does with the dyad, the child begins to experience moments of safely relaxing and having someone provide for her needs. Theraplay's parallel process of working with the caregiver, including meeting that caregiver's needs, allows the caregiver to experience these moments of calm and worth also. Both caregiver and child come to believe in the caregiver's ability to learn and change. Some children and caregivers are slower than others to accept good touch as a soothing and enjoyable experience. While being sensitive to the individual's need to build tolerance and then comfort with nurture, it is imperative also to be brave with our proximity, our affirmations, our use of every opportunity to give even slight moments of good touch, so that those who have been neglected, berated, threatened and hurt can know the exhilaration of feeling accepted, valued and touchable. This is not a cognitive but visceral communication!

5. Use Theraplay engagement, challenge and playfulness to provide the impetus for change

The three remaining dimensions weave together to create potential motivation for change through the messages provided in new experiences of safe play, social interaction and teamwork.

Table 10.3: Engagement

The message of engagement for the child	The message of engagement for the caregiver
You are not alone. You are safe. Your caregiver wants to be with you. Your caregiver sees and hears you. Your caregiver understands you.	You have the power to connect with your child with your voice, eyes, face, touch and movement. Your gentle social connection makes your child feel safer. You can create a special "dance" of interaction with your child that no one else has. You can understand your child, which helps him understand himself and other people. You can help your child learn the give and take of healthy relationships.

The *engagement* dimension provides an experience of shared safe connection and joy, both of which are uncertain or absent within families with DV patterns. Consider the power of Theraplay's messages within the *engagement* dimension for a caregiver and child who have felt alone, unsafe, disconnected and powerless to do anything about it! As we guide the dyadic activities and interact with the caregiver, while displaying the warmth, kindness and empathy that we want the caregiver to have with their child, the caregiver also experiences the same messages as the child gets from engagement. This experience can provide the impetus for life-changing new choices. Negative experiences keep us stuck in unhealthy situations and outlooks, because we feel helpless; positive experiences energize us towards change, because we begin to see possibilities.

Children affected by DV often have difficulty focusing on the here and now; they are instead preoccupied with either revisiting past traumas or anticipating future ones. This can be just as true for the caregiver. Because traumatizing messages and actions have been ongoing (perhaps in the caregiver's early life as well) and are being repeatedly reinforced by DV family patterns, change is often a slow and careful process of reconstruction towards believing that "I *can* trust, feel, talk about things, and do things differently." Through Theraplay's repeated experiences of acceptance, patient guidance and small "moments of meeting," we begin to construct capacity for the caregiver and child to be truly present with each other and to experience the enjoyment of each other.

The *challenge* dimension of Theraplay offers repeated small opportunities to try something new and experience success, both in accomplishing the task and doing it as a team. Within a system of DV, maintaining the status quo—"not rocking the boat" and risking emotional or physical attack—feels safer and thus becomes the goal. So trying new things and expecting success and enjoyment can be difficult, perhaps even scary. Since Theraplay's *challenge* involves supporting caregivers and children as they try something new, they gain a growing awareness of self-efficacy. Challenge activities are always within the zone of proximal development (Vygotsky, 1978), that is, tasks that are difficult for a child to master alone but can be done with an adult's supportive guidance.

Table 10.4: Challenge

The message of challenge for the child	The message of challenge for the caregiver
You are strong and competent.	You can help your child feel strong and capable.
You are capable of making good things happen.	You can help your child grow and develop skills.
You can accomplish something that is a bit difficult with your caregiver's help.	You can learn what to expect your child can do.
	You can be a partner with your child.
	You can discover ways to give positive feedback.
	You can enjoy your child's accomplishments.

Self-efficacy is about a person's belief in their own ability to successfully accomplish something they decide to do. The lack of this belief, and the resulting anxiety or shame, often lead to resistance from caregiver or child or both within Theraplay sessions. So we practitioners must thoughtfully plan for how we can deliver these messages, not just in words, but through interactive experiences with the caregiver and with the dyad. We make our expectations realistic, then we acknowledge and cheer each small step. All the messages in our complex trauma chart (Lindaman, 2015) aim to promote self-efficacy—that is, a new sense of being able to do things when I have been told I cannot. Yet, there is an "aha" experience within *engagement*'s surprising moments of connection, *challenge*'s empowering moments of accomplishment, and *play*'s joyful moments of fun, which can ignite and fuel the desire to change.

Play in Theraplay parallels the bonding interactions of a healthy caregiver and child.

Table 10.5: Play

The message of play for the child	The message of play for the caregiver
You are fun to be with.	You can bring joy and hope to your child.
There is joy in relationships.	Playing together helps your child manage positive and negative feelings.
	Your play shows your child how to interact with others.
	Joyful play creates a strong connection and good feelings.

These playful interactions communicate safety and reduce stress while promoting learning and well-being (Purvis, Cross & Sunshine, 2007). Yet, play often is unfamiliar and perhaps even uncomfortable for the caregiver and child who have experienced the constraints of DV. If they seem resistant to the idea or the experience of play, we may be tempted to avoid playfulness as being too dissonant with the seriousness of their life experience. If they seem simply unsure, or if they are compliant, we may bring in lots of play with hopes of "just bringing joy" to this dyad. However, our best approach is to move at a sensitive pace while bravely leading in *small* steps of playfulness. Being both sensitive and brave requires three components:

- We plan well before sessions.

- We reflect well after sessions.

- Within the session we present play in an attuned way.

To successfully draw a child and caregiver into play, we become the interesting object of focus as we do something gently surprising that invites participation; for example, noticing body parts that are wiggly or still, showing how fingertips and a thumb can make a "puppy print" in Playdoh. Also, we are down on the floor at their level and ready to interact using familiar though unlikely play items (newspaper, cotton balls, a scarf). For children affected by DV, this is so different from the adults they are used to, and it piques their interest and paves the way for moments of joy, then hope and then trust.

Caregivers who have seen their child fearful, withdrawn, vigilant or angry much of the time may suddenly see a spark of interest and joy as we draw the child/dyad into playful interaction. The caregiver may feel the enticement of play themselves, and they see interactions that they could do with their child. Those moments create a glimmer of hope for the caregiver too. As Theraplay practitioners, we have the opportunity to demonstrate and to guide the caregiver into the reality of the last message in the chart: "Joyful play creates a strong connection and good feelings." A glimmer at times seems too small and faint. Yet, think of a campfire on a cold evening: its source is a single spark, even if repeated attempts are needed before it catches flame or if conditions dampen it and we must begin again. This is an apt analogy for our work with clients from DV, especially if the caregiver grew up in DV or is living with apprehension currently. So, we now have circled back to the need for working first with the non-offending caregiver, like preparing the wood for the campfire so that the flame will catch!

 ## CASE ILLUSTRATION

A mother (Judy) with two young children, six-year-old Luke and four-year-old Cindy, was referred to me by a colleague after Judy's husband, Pete, was arrested for domestic battery. In her call to me, she described marital conflict beginning soon after the birth of her first child. She and Pete often disagreed about money, responsibilities and decisions about the children. She was frightened and unsure what to do about recent escalations in the conflict.

INTAKE

I began by focusing on Judy's current experience and gathered a bit of her history about her marriage and her own childhood experiences. Judy described her own parents as strict and always busy working: her dad at his job and her mom taking care of the house and the children. They expected the children to be good, do what they were told, and work hard in school. They were proud of their son, the oldest child, because he was very good at baseball and made good grades. Judy noted that he often got away with mercilessly teasing the girls and blaming them if anything went wrong. Her older sister, the middle child, got frequent spankings for "back talk" whenever she "told on" her brother or questioned her parents' decisions. Judy described herself as working very hard to be good and never calling attention to herself. She remembered her parents quarreling off and on throughout her childhood, then avoiding each other until things "blew over"; the children would go off by themselves until the tension went down. She didn't know if or how her parents ever resolved issues.

Judy saw herself as a hard worker, able to work well with others at her job. Some friends introduced her to Pete, and she loved her husband's strength and decisiveness in the beginning. Things seemed okay until she gave birth to Luke and became busy with his care. He had colic and cried a lot, which angered Pete. As time went on, she began to feel that she could never do anything right at home. Pete was consistently unhappy and critical of her. Judy told of experiencing persistent criticism, accusations and blame if she expressed a different opinion or addressed any problems. However, she denied past physical harm from Pete and was shocked when he became aggressive, grabbed her arms and shook her, then shoved her aside as he left the home in anger. The force of his shove caused Judy to fall heavily, breaking her arm and hitting her head. The children were terrified. Judy felt fearful for their safety if she said nothing but feared Pete's reaction if she reported the incident. When she went to the emergency room with the children, medical personnel saw the need to report the battery to the police, who located Pete and arrested him. A court date was set and he was instructed to live with a local family member until then.

After listening and empathizing with the fear she and the children must have felt, I shared with her a list of personal relational rights, which actually are personal *needs*: for example, "The right to goodwill from the other," "The right to be heard by the other and to be responded to with courtesy," "The right to have one's own feelings and experiences acknowledged as real," "The right to be respectfully asked rather than ordered" (Evans, 2010, p.122). Some of these were new to Judy and she indicated that many of these were not respected in her marriage. We set another appointment to discuss this further and to explore her own goals and expectations for family life.

SECOND INDIVIDUAL SESSION WITH JUDY

Judy came with more questions this time after thinking about the list of personal rights. I shared more information with her about the cycle that can develop within a marriage when problems are never fully discussed and resolved (often described as the cycle of violence). Tension mounts and leads to behaviors and words that spark quarrels, anger, bad feelings and even verbal or physical abuse. If the parties are unable or unwilling to learn skills to calm themselves down and communicate about the problems underneath the tension, then the cycle continues and often worsens. We discussed the eroding and triggering effects this pattern leads to for both adults and children. We also discussed the reasons why it can be difficult for a woman to decide when to stay and when to leave her partner.

Judy began to reveal more aspects of the conflict that had occurred and described effects she saw on her children. While Cindy was very sweet and quiet, and enjoyed playing with other children in her pre-kindergarten class, she had become more shy and even clingy at times. Judy's bigger concern was for Luke's behaviors: a pattern of headaches and nightmares, plus quick frustration with many tasks, leading to tears and belligerence, especially if he felt criticized in any way. These behaviors angered Pete, who then became stern, critical and punitive with Luke. Pete criticized Judy for her parenting style with Luke and often left the home in a huff. Later he would feel bad, bring gifts to Luke and apologize for getting angry, but the pattern repeated consistently. Judy felt it must be very confusing to Luke. She would then "baby" Luke to make up for Pete's harshness, but she saw that her responses were not helping with Luke's behaviors. We discussed Judy's goals for her family, options for intervention, and I gave her some information to read and consider before our next appointment.

THIRD INDIVIDUAL SESSION WITH JUDY

Judy informed me that Pete had been persistently calling and texting her, alternating between pleading for her to drop the charges and threatening her when she refused. She considered changing the locks, but still felt unsafe, so she had removed herself and the children from the home to a safe place. She hesitantly revealed that Pete had attended an anger management class in the past but that the physical threats never truly ceased. The reading material was showing her that the verbal abuse was more harmful than she had realized and had given her a sense of her children's need for therapy too. I suggested that we began with a MIM assessment for her and Luke, since his behaviors were of most concern, then we would meet to discuss a plan for treatment. I waited to see the outcome of the arrest and separation before considering when and in what way to include Pete.

MIM

In the MIM, Judy was gentle, playful and able to engage Luke in play during squeaky animals. Both displayed mutual enjoyment and moments of synchrony. Judy seemed a bit tentative at first, yet nurturing in the lotion task and feeding task, and Luke readily accepted both. In the teach task, Mom tried to teach Luke to fold paper into an airplane. Luke was excited at first but quickly became agitated when he found the folding a bit difficult, so he crumpled the paper, became tearful and told Mom, "I can't do it!" Judy's face showed both surprise and concern; she began to reassure him that everything is hard on the first try and they could go slowly, one fold at a time. This encouragement allowed Luke to begin again and complete the airplane. Although he still showed disappointment that his did not fly as well as Mom's, Mom praised his efforts and assured him they would keep practicing at home. At the close of the MIM, when Mom was asked which activity she thought Luke liked best and least, Judy showed distress about Luke's experience with the folding and blamed herself for picking something too difficult.

MIM PARENT FEEDBACK

From the three individual sessions with Judy, I saw that in the conflictual family of her childhood she had learned to accept a position of powerlessness when mistreated, to be cautious of speaking up, to work hard to please and to quietly balance out negatives in order to stay safe.

These might be obstacles for the Theraplay work and would need to be addressed in parent sessions. However, in the MIM, I observed that Judy saw and had empathy for her child's distress, plus she was able to emotionally support her child. Thus, for this feedback session, my goal was to lend support to Judy and to empower her to be a safe base for Luke by affirming her capacities as seen in the MIM.

I showed Judy the nice interactions of the squeaky animals, with her comfortable closeness and her playful leading so that Luke could relax and enjoy the mutual play. Then I introduced the clip of the teach task by letting her know that I saw their distress in the moment, but that I wanted her to see the positive things she had done to help Luke.

Judy agreed that it had been distressing and said she did not recall any positives. As we watched the sequence, I asked what she had experienced at that time. She blamed herself for choosing something too hard for Luke and causing him to feel incompetent. I wondered with her about her own feelings as a child and as an adult, receiving criticism with no one affirming her positive qualities and helping her to repair, and how those might affect her view of her ability now to help her own children. After I pointed out her encouraging responses that helped Luke to keep trying, she was able to look at the video clip with new eyes.

My messages to Judy were that:

- her own feeling of powerlessness actually made the moment feel more significant than anything else in the MIM, when in fact it was one brief moment and she had done a good job of responding to Luke's distress by encouraging him

- her own sense of inadequacy hid from her the positive things that she had actually done to repair Luke's insecurity

- a child being distressed and a parent responding with reassurance is actually the necessary process for Luke to become able to try things, make mistakes and learn to try again without feeling bad about himself.

Reflecting the positive capacities that Judy demonstrated was essential to her preparation for working on relational repair with her son in the Theraplay.

CAREGIVER DEMONSTRATION SESSION

This session is especially important for a caregiver from domestic violence because it affords an opportunity for the caregiver to experience and learn about the four dimensions and the playfulness that work together to foster a sense of safety, sense of self and sense of being valued/respected that is difficult to develop within a conflictual family system. It also gives you the practitioner the opportunity to learn more about the caregiver's own needs—from childhood and/or from the more recent family violence—so that you can decide whether more preparation and additional resources will be needed.

Judy's strength was that she was beginning to see what she had missed and wanted to learn how to give that to her children. We met individually several more times to prepare her before beginning dyadic sessions: exploring what she wanted for herself and her children, her fears about supporting herself and her children if she left Pete, and her concerns about sharing caregiving with him. I gave her more information to read between sessions to address her concerns. We spent additional time practicing the Theraplay activities in order to meet her own emotional-social needs and to help her understand how the activities could help her child. As we worked together, I saw her starting to accept herself as a "normal" person with both strengths and areas for growth. She began to feel some anger at her caregivers and Pete for the criticism and blame they had given her and the emotional support they had not given. While acknowledging her right to feel angry, we worked on moving her focus from a focus on her caregivers and husband (which had always disempowered her) to a focus on growth for her and her children. She began to trust me as a supportive resource and became eager to learn better interventions with Luke. She would still need more support in considering options for the future and in practicing new assertiveness skills, but I saw her developing the foundation to be a safe base for her children. We could begin Theraplay work, moving slowly, while having more frequent caregiver sessions to support her own growth.

TREATMENT SESSIONS
Sessions 1–3 with Luke and Mom

In order to provide a sense of safety within the therapy setting for both caregiver and child, *structure* and *engagement* were the initial dimensions of focus. I focused on predictability, organization and a rhythmic and calm pace, making sure that I moved along in a way that allowed Luke and Judy to anticipate my next move. In addition, I paid attention to my own social engagement system cues (face, voice, head and shoulder movements) in order to provide the calm, playful interaction which would signal safety and enable Luke to engage (Porges, 2018). Mom was present from the beginning, to provide a sense of safety and to be the joint participant and learner who could show approval of new activities and could do physical contact. I carefully guided the interaction without moving in too close, too fast.

Luke loved trains, so I used this interest for my entrance activity. I asked him to make the train whistle sounds, and in follow-the-leader style we used our arms for the wheel movements and choo-chooed from the door, around the perimeter of the room until the rhythmic movements had established a sense of playfulness and soothing pace, while giving Luke a chance to survey the room and feel more at ease. Judy and Luke seemed relaxed as we sat after the playful rhythmic movement.

We did a structured check-up, noticing "parts" of Luke that could move: his eyebrows, his fingers, his bending elbows, his feet. I included Judy in this check-up by seeing if her parts moved the same way. This helped them to look at each other and to laugh at times, especially when I checked Mom's elbows and made a squeaky sound as I moved each. I then showed Mom a sound that Luke had, as I popped my cheeks gently and then gently helped Luke to pop his own puffed cheeks. I next asked Judy to notice any special spots or "owies" that we needed to be careful of during our activities. There were none, so I counted his fingers on each hand and guided Mom to do "This Little Piggy" with his fingers, naming foods he liked for one hand and activities he enjoyed for the other. (Mom was well prepared since we practiced this in our parent demonstration session.) When Mom named ten items, Luke smiled and leaned into her for a hug. While Luke was experiencing being seen, heard and valued, Mom was learning the very basics of being able to help her child feel calmer, safer and cared for.

Structure and co-regulation continued with a carefully guided bubble pop: Mom and Luke clapping a few bubbles with hands, Mom holding Luke's feet to clap a few, then Luke popping one bubble with a finger of his choice, a toe, a cheek, an ear lobe, while Mom wiped off any wetness on each part. To promote Luke's self-awareness in these early sessions, I used such activities as measuring, lotion prints of his and Mom's hand, hand stack, blow me over/pull me up, and a version of the copy me game in which we stood and used big muscle movement with some start-stop-notice of poses and ending with standing stiff as a board and hanging soft as a noodle. I guided the activities in ways that provided clear direction, easy pace, grounding proprioceptive input and rhythmic movement that felt calming and safe to both. Judy later told me that she had not realized until then that she had missed doing these pleasurable activities in the past because of her focus on getting things done in order to keep peace in the home.

Judy let me know that for a while, when the children missed their old house, they would all talk about different pets they might get now, since neither she nor they had been allowed to have one. Luke brought that conversation into one of the sessions several times. So to bring the focus from talk (cognitive) to being present together (relational), I included a very structured form of the funny animal kisses activity. This added a bit of nurture in a way that seemed fun to Luke; it became one of their favorite bedtime rituals. It is helpful to blend the dimensions (e.g., doing *structure* in an engaging or nurturing way or *nurture* in a structured way) in order to maintain the safe, organized, predictable feel for parent and child while they still experience the connection and care that lead to mutual enjoyment. Looking again at the complex trauma chart, the messages of structure, engagement and nurture were already beginning to settle in at the end of dyadic session 3.

Regarding Dad

After the individual work, then the start of the Theraplay work, plus several ongoing support sessions, Judy felt ready to file for divorce and for sole custody of the children. In light of Pete's ongoing threatening harassment of her, in spite of her being granted an Order of Protection, the divorce proceedings went through quickly and Judy was awarded sole custody. Visitation for Pete was on hold until he completed the required treatment program for domestic abuse offenders. Continuation of the Theraplay treatment for Luke with his mom was included in the recommendations of the decree.

Sessions 4–6 with Luke and Mom

I maintained close *structure*, plus added more of the *engagement* activities (e.g., hand claps and passing funny faces), and more intimate *nurture* from Mom to Luke (e.g., lotion massage of hands/arms/feet, airplane, blanket swing/wrap, weather report, special ways of feeding). Judy and Luke began to talk about activities they were doing at home that helped them feel calmer and less grumpy and made bedtimes more relaxed. We discussed in parent sessions the goals of the Theraplay activities that we were doing; as Judy experienced their impact on Luke and on herself, she understood how the activities offered new ways to co-regulate Luke's emotions through movement, rhythm and touch. Luke frequently wanted me to see a new way he and Mom were doing their handshake or copy me or a new clapping game. This parent and child were beginning to internalize the Theraplay messages identified in the complex trauma chart! Mom was learning that "Your gentle social connection helps your child feel safer" and "You can figure out the best way to calm and soothe your child." Similarly, Luke was learning that "You are not alone. Your parent sees and hears you…and understands you. Your parent can help you feel better."

Sessions 7–9 with Luke and Mom

As Judy became stronger emotionally and relationally, Luke's attachment to her became more secure. Now when Luke had a "meltdown" moment, Mom better understood what he was feeling and knew some things to help calm him. I began to add more challenge activities to build Luke's ability to move through the tension of uncertainty so he could experience those moments of success that led to competence and confidence. Mom was excited to learn more playful ways she could support this process. In this way, both were gaining a growing sense of "personal power," which victims of family violence need so much but do not have the opportunity to develop. I created "Olympic steps," to promote a sense of self-efficacy for Luke and to help Judy see how important her attunement and affirmation were in supporting Luke's efforts. After enthusiastically measuring Luke's height and wingspan, I eased into challenge by measuring a succession of his steps and jumps: a "normal" step, a "giant" step, and then three separate broad jumps from the same starting point and marked with a sticker or masking tape at the heel of the step. Each time, I guided Luke back to the starting point and encouraged him to see each increase in his progress. For the second jump, I encouraged Mom to cheer for Luke and then asked: "Did you know, Mom, how powerful your cheering is?" I asked Luke if he was too tired or would like another try. He was eager to do it again, to get additional notice and praise from Mom! Luke felt empowered as he focused his energy and saw progress with each effort. His mom felt empowered that she could help her child achieve through the encouragement of simple affirmation.

Paper punch, using two fingers held straight together instead of a fist, really made Luke feel strong. Blow me over, push me over/pull me up, karate chop and active start-and-stop versions of copy me all offer good opportunities to build the child's *sense of self* (which body part do I need to use?), *self-efficacy* (look what I did!) and *personal power* (I can decide to do/stop doing something and make it happen and then celebrate it!). Teaching the parent to celebrate the child's *efforts* rather than just *accomplishments* helps the parent not only to really see their child but also to feel competent in building the capacities of the child. Again, the experiences build the messages from the chart into the being of the child and the parent.

Session 10 with Luke and Mom

Treatment session 10 was our final session before Judy began to move into some new directions of growth: new job training, a new support group with other women recovering from the effects of DV, and moving in with a family member who could help with childcare. We had a party with some of Luke's favorite snacks and activities, and his sister, Cindy, came with Luke and Mom to enjoy the fun. Cindy seemed to have lost much of her shyness as Mom used her new knowledge and skills at home with both children. Judy did continue in monthly support sessions during the following year and seemed to be maintaining her progress even through some difficult situations.

A final note about Theraplay for families who have experienced DV

An extra piece of planning in working with families who have experienced DV is to think about things that could come up within the system and try to plan with the caregiver a structured way to handle them. One example is children who have visitation with the offending caregiver (usually the case if that caregiver has not directly abused the child, physically or sexually, and does not seem to pose a threat to the child); the child may want to teach their non-involved caregiver some of the "games" they are learning in session. This can backfire on the child. One way this happens is that a non-attending caregiver learns the activities, perhaps reluctantly, and then does them in a non-Theraplay manner which could be emotionally hurtful to the child. Another way is that the non-attending caregiver criticizes and devalues both the therapy and the caregiver who is involved in the therapy. Remember that an abusing caregiver can act very differently in and out of session. This becomes a double negative for the child, who feels belittled and even shamed for their enthusiasm and who also hears more negatives about the non-abusing caregiver.

Since it usually is not safe for the child to express true feelings, she ends up having to act the part of agreeing with the abusive caregiver or aligning with that caregiver and no longer taking a chance on true participation in the Theraplay. It is helpful to speak about this at the end of the first Theraplay session if the child seems to be enjoying the activities. You can simply say that sometimes children go to visit their other caregiver and want to teach the games they've enjoyed, but it's better for each caregiver to learn them here, where the therapist can guide things to work well: for example, "I'll talk with your dad about coming on some of the days you are visiting him so he can learn the activities too. Until then, we'll play them here, and Mom will be learning them so you two can do them together when you are with her. I'll let you know when I've talked with Dad and when he's coming in, okay?" If I am able to work with that caregiver, I try to be very clear that my job is to help the child have the best possible relationship with each caregiver, because that is in the best interest of the child.

I have discussed the preparatory work that often needs to be done with a non-offending caregiver who has been affected by DV. In my case example, I was able to work with the mom to sufficiently build her capacities and confidence so that she could participate as a safe attachment figure for her child. If she had not been able to work through the effects of the DV to take on that role, then I would have needed to explore other potential attachment figures within the family system, or perhaps use a different therapeutic modality and include select Theraplay activities to address social-emotional skills for the child's school or daycare needs. In cultures where extended family relationships are strong, other family members may be able to fill the gap.

Even when Theraplay is your primary modality, you should be prepared to provide opportunities for the child to talk about their experiences of the abuse in the presence of a safe, supportive person. I've worked with children who display aggression or somatic symptoms of stress before or after a visit with the offending caregiver. I've included some sessions, or partial sessions, that allow opportunities to talk while drawing, using my sand tray, building with Lego or playing board games. I work at being very careful not to intrude with lots of questions and not to reflect anything negative about the offending caregiver. Once I've built trust through the Theraplay work, I've found that a child may reveal many more of their feelings and their coping mechanisms than I ever expected. The most helpful responses in this case are simple ones: "It makes sense to me that you would feel that way" and "Adults can be really confusing sometimes, can't they?" These seem to support a child's experience! These talk times not only help the child release inner pressure in a safe way, but also help the non-offending caregiver not to get caught in the middle, either minimizing their child's concerns or getting upset with the offending caregiver and perhaps being seen as alienating the child from the other caregiver. Once the child has released sufficient inner pressure for the moment, they often seek some Theraplay activities to help rejoin with their caregiver before leaving.

Lastly, when working with this population, you need to learn all that you can about the systemic patterns of DV, the mindset of a reactive or controlling abuser (Bancroft, 2002), the effects on the partner and the children who witness and experience abusive patterns of behavior (including the IWM and the survival thinking that leads to the partner and children's responses), the information they do not know, and the skills they need to learn. The dyad in my case example made a fairly rapid change due to the readiness and basic capacities of the mom. This is not the case in many of these family situations! This process can be difficult and discouraging for the practitioner as well as for the client for at least three reasons:

1. Usually there will be frequent steps backward during the journey forward.

2. The messages of the abusive system are deeply engrained and may be consistently reinforced outside the therapy sessions.

3. The fear of revealing information leads to tendencies to hide things or to react with avoidance, anger or compliance, which can foster countertransference in the practitioner. However, when we understand the factors that keep families caught in patterns of DV, we will not so easily lose patience with those who have difficulty getting unstuck.

The references at the end of this chapter can help you begin this journey.

Questions for reflection and continued learning

1. What are the four significant characteristics of emotional abuse?

2. What are three factors within domestic violence that could present difficulty for Theraplay intervention with dyads who have experienced DV?

3. Can you identify at least four ways in which Theraplay can have a positive impact on a dyad that has experienced DV?

References

Bancroft, L. (2002). *Why Does He Do That? Inside the Minds of Angry and Controlling Men*. New York, NY: The Berkley Publishing Group.

Bancroft, L. (2004). *When Dad Hurts Mom*. New York, NY: Penguin Group.

Dugan, M. & Hock, R. (2006). *It's My Life Now: Starting Over After an Abusive Relationship or Domestic Violence*. New York, NY: Routledge.

Evans, P. (2010). *The Verbally Abusive Relationship*. Avon, MA: Adams Media.

Gates, D. (2010). "Using Theraplay to help families with patterns of domestic violence." *The Theraplay Institute Newsletter*.

Lindaman, S. (2015). "How the Dimensions of Theraplay Meet the Needs of Children and Caregivers." Handout of The Theraplay Institute.

Meyer, S. & Frost, A. (2019). *Domestic and Family Violence*. Abingdon, Oxfordshire, UK: Routledge.

National Center on Domestic and Sexual Violence. (2016). *Domestic Violence Personalized Safety Plan*. Retrieved from www.ncdsv.org/images/DV_Safety_Plan.pdf.

National Child Traumatic Stress Network. (2019). *Intimate Partner Violence*. Retrieved from www.nctsn.org/what-is-child-trauma/trauma-types/intimate-partner-violence.

Perry, B.D. (2006). "Applying Principles of Neurodevelopment to Clinical Work with Maltreated and Traumatized Children: The Neurosequential Model of Therapeutics." In N.B. Webb (ed.) *Social Work Practice with Children and Families: Working with Traumatized Youth in Child Welfare* (pp.27–52). New York, NY: Guilford Press.

Porges, S. (2018). *Face to Face Social Engagement* [Video file]. Retrieved from www.youtube.com/watch?v=lxS3bv32-UY.

Purvis, K., Cross, D. & Sunshine, W.L. (2007). *The Connected Child*. New York, NY: McGraw-Hill.

Vygotsky, L.S. (1978). *Mind in Society: The Development of Higher Psychological Processes*. Cambridge, MA: Harvard University Press.

Walker, L. (2017). *The Battered Woman Syndrome* (fourth edition). New York, NY: Springer Publishing Company.

Chapter 11

Adapting Theraplay for Affirmative Intervention with LGBTQ Families

Lauren C. Smithee

Introduction

This chapter discusses Theraplay intervention with LGBTQ families. While there is an incredible amount of diversity among LGBTQ people, within this chapter, "LGBTQ" is used as an umbrella term for individuals with sexual and/or gender minority identities (e.g., lesbian, gay, bisexual, transgender, queer). As practitioners intervene with LGBTQ families, it is important to be mindful of other facets of identity that impact family members' social locations (positioning in society based on identity) such as race, ethnicity, socio-economic status, and ability. However, this chapter will focus on adapting Theraplay for the needs of LGBTQ families specifically. While this chapter focuses on LGBTQ families, practitioners ought to use an intersectional lens to consider how the social location of each family member impacts their experience in society, as well as how the practitioner's social location impacts the therapy process.

Key points

The reader will become familiar with the following key points for Theraplay with LGBTQ families:

1. The practitioner must consider the impact of minority stress (i.e., the stress that comes with belonging to a minority group) on

attachment bonds. An understanding of LGBTQ stigma combined with affirmative practices in Theraplay can help practitioners strengthen attachment bonds.

2. LGBTQ affirmative language is critical to promote safety and development of therapeutic alliance (see the Glossary of LGBTQ terms at the end of the chapter).

3. Working with LGBTQ families may necessitate additional caregiver consultation sessions to (a) process feelings of loss, confusion and fear about their child's future and/or to process caregiver experiences with minority stress, and to (b) provide psychoeducation about sexuality and gender.

4. Special attention to the nurture and engagement dimensions may be most important to promote loving, accepting interactions between caregiver and child, and to communicate unconditional love, in light of the impact of minority stress on attachment.

5. Since familial reactions to LGBTQ identity disclosure may be an attachment wound, the practitioner should assess for caregiver reactions to disclosure and the impact on the family.

Impact of minority stress and internalized stigma on psychological health and attachment

- *LGBTQ youth.* Research consistently indicates that LGBTQ populations experience disproportionate rates of rejection, discrimination, harassment and violence compared with heterosexual and cisgender populations (Centers for Disease Control and Prevention, 2017; DeCamp & Bakken, 2016; Meyer, Teylan & Schwartz, 2015; Muehlenkamp *et al.*, 2015; Pitoňák, 2017; Smithee, Sumner & Bean, 2019). This often contributes to a devalued sense of self and higher rates of depression, anxiety, isolation and suicidal ideation among LGBTQ populations compared with heterosexual and cisgender individuals (Centers for Disease Control and Prevention, 2017; DeCamp & Bakken, 2016; House *et al.*, 2011; Meyer, 2003; Pitoňák, 2017; Smithee *et al.*, 2019). LGBTQ youth are especially vulnerable to experiencing minority stress due to their relative lack of agency, access to resources, and independence compared with adults. This is especially true for transgender and gender diverse (TGD) youth, who ultimately need parental permission for legal and/or medical transition (Drescher & Byne, 2012; Steensma *et al.*, 2011).

- *Children of LGBTQ caregivers.* The detrimental effects of exposure to LGBTQ stigma does not only extend to LGBTQ youth, but to children of LGBTQ caregivers. While research has consistently found no significant differences in the well-being of children of heterosexual and cisgender caregivers compared with children of LGBTQ caregivers, social stigma negatively impacts both LGBTQ caregivers and their children (Manning, Fettro & Lamidi, 2014; Trub *et al.*, 2016). Experience of transphobic and/or homophobic stigma within LGBTQ families is associated with adverse effects on well-being, including lower self-esteem, parenting insecurity, greater feelings of isolation, and identity conflicts (Manning *et al.*, 2014; Trub *et al.*, 2016). LGBTQ caregivers are often subject to minority stress, especially within the heteronormative sphere of childrearing, and can experience social exclusion.

Considering the pervasive impacts of internalized stigma and minority stress on well-being, it is no surprise that experienced discrimination negatively impacts familial attachment bonds (Levy, Russon & Diamond, 2016; Rosario *et al.*, 2014). Experiences with internalized stigma and minority stress can impact LGBTQ youths' inner working model of self ("I am unlovable," "My LGBTQ family is shameful") and others ("I cannot trust others to be accepting," "Others will only judge my family"). In contrast, growing up within a secure attachment bond can help buffer against interpersonal and societal experiences with LGBTQ stigma (Levy *et al.*, 2016; Rosario *et al.*, 2014). Research has found that secure familial attachment is protective against exposure to transphobia and homophobia (Levy *et al.*, 2016; Rosario *et al.*, 2014; Trub *et al.*, 2016). For example, feeling safe to communicate about one's experiences and gain support in the face of potential obstacles such as LGBTQ-focused bullying is tremendously protective. Considering the importance of attachment in buffering against internalized stigma, Theraplay may be especially impactful in promoting well-being in LGBTQ families.

Adaptations and considerations when intervening with LGBTQ families

This chapter integrates Theraplay with principles of affirmative therapy for best intervention with LGBTQ families. By employing the following, the practitioner can facilitate increased feelings of safety within the caregiver-child bond and coach caregivers to promote a more positive internal working model within themselves and their child.

Therapist education

Before applying these recommendations, the practitioner must have a firm understanding not only of Theraplay intervention but also of (a) the differences between sexual orientation, gender identity, biological sex and gender expression, (b) the unique experiences of LGBTQ youth with identity formation, and (c) principles of affirmative practice with LGBTQ youth and families. It is also important to know that despite sexual and gender minority identities being under the same umbrella term (LGBTQ), the experiences of individuals with these identity markers differ.

While many LGBTQ individuals have similarities in their experiences with coming out to others, the LGBTQ population is not a homogenous group of people. For example, TGD youth often cope with additional stressors compared to cisgender sexual minority youth, such as internalized transphobia, gender dysphoria and social, legal and/or medical transitioning (Smithee *et al.*, 2019). As such, the practitioner may hold even greater power and responsibility when working with TGD youth, since they often require a diagnosis of gender dysphoria and/or letters of support from a mental health practitioner before medical interventions can occur (e.g., puberty suppression and/or cross-sex hormones). Before intervening with this population, the practitioner must educate themselves with the WPATH Standards of Care (World Professional Association for Transgender Health, 2018) for ethical practice. Furthermore, these identities are not mutually exclusive. An individual could identify either as a sexual minority (lesbian, pansexual, etc.) or a gender minority (trans man, non-binary, agender, etc.), or as both (e.g., a lesbian trans woman). The practitioner must disregard their assumptions and ask LGBTQ youth (and LGBTQ caregivers) for their preferred name and pronouns, especially if the client is out as a gender minority.

Communicating safety and support through inclusive language

When using Theraplay with LGBTQ families, it is also critical to communicate support through inclusive and affirmative language. While Theraplay is focused on creating experiences of interpersonal connection and attunement within the room, the practitioner can integrate affirmative language into these sequences to increase safety and the impact of these interactions. LGBTQ families often experience microaggressions or even overt aggressions regularly, so even small, caring interactions such as a warm, affirming greeting to the family can help create a welcoming, safe refuge. Similarly, the practitioner should intentionally use inclusive language within speech and intake forms and assessments. Simple changes in gendered and heteronormative language such as referring to parents as "caregivers" instead of "mother" and "father" can be powerful. Exposure to heteronormative language can be experienced as a microaggression and decrease feelings of safety needed for deeper attachment work (Bernal & Coolhart, 2012; Coolhart, 2012; Harvey & Stone Fish, 2015).

Most importantly, it is critical for the practitioner to honor the language their LGBTQ clients use to describe their identities. The language LGBTQ youth and adults choose to describe their identities is often deeply symbolic of their sense of self and warrants utmost respect and affirmation. The practitioner is responsible for modeling the appropriate use of names and pronouns (i.e., the youth's chosen name and pronouns rather than name/pronouns used at birth) for caregivers if youth are TGD. The practitioner may even consider utilizing Theraplay interventions that allow for the practitioner to purposefully use the child's chosen name and pronouns to demonstrate respect and affirmation of LGBTQ identities. This strengthens the therapeutic alliance and models ways in which parents can show affirmation through everyday interactions.

Caregiver support and psychoeducation
Caregiver support

When conducting Theraplay with LGBTQ youth, promoting sequences of interpersonal connection becomes complicated by caregiver understanding and acceptance of sexual orientation and gender identity. Practitioners who implement Theraplay with LGBTQ families are advised to integrate principles of affirmative therapy into their clinical practice to facilitate an environment in which safety and acceptance can flourish (Bernal & Coolhart, 2012; Coolhart, 2012; Harvey & Stone Fish, 2015). The practitioner must balance their alliances with both the youth and their caregivers, while simultaneously fostering empathy for each member's experiences. Caregivers of LGBTQ youth often experience loss, confusion and fear for their child's future, and the practitioner must provide an emotionally safe environment during consultation sessions to help caregivers process these feelings (Coolhart, 2012; Norwood, 2013). Helping members process confusion and grief surrounding their experiences while nurturing LGBTQ identities is essential to promote the emergence of more positive connections. Similarly, LGBTQ caregivers may potentially need additional consultation sessions to process their experiences with minority stress and for the practitioner to offer support in light of potential experiences with rejection from others within their community or broadly, especially since parenthood is often laced with heteronormative assumptions. The number of caregiver support sessions needed will greatly differ based on the individual needs of each family.

Caregiver psychoeducation

In addition to offering consultation sessions to support LGBTQ caregivers and/or caregivers of LGBTQ youth, Theraplay must also incorporate psychoeducation about sexuality and gender identity. Just as the practitioner uses psychoeducation to teach about the dimensions of Theraplay, emotional regulation and attachment theory, the practitioner must also teach caregivers about the current research on supporting the mental health of LGBTQ youth (Bernal & Coolhart, 2012; Coolhart, 2012; Harvey & Stone Fish, 2015). Knowing how powerful family support and connection is in buffering against internalized stigma can empower and motivate caregivers (Ryan, 2009). Finally, when working with caregivers struggling to accept their child's identity, the practitioner might delay direct participation of the caregiver in sessions, due to the potential for further attachment wounds (e.g., caregivers using incorrect name or pronouns for the TGD child). The practitioner should carefully frame a decision to delay caregiver involvement around the status of psychoeducation on the impact of minority stress on attachment. Until the caregivers have processed their reactions to their child's identity, therapy may progress more quickly with the caregivers initially observing and learning how to better attune to their child.

Attention to engagement and nurture dimensions

While the practitioner will attend to nurture, engagement, structure and challenge to varying degrees, based on the needs of each child and caregiver, LGBTQ families may need additional experiences with engagement and nurture. Especially for LGBTQ youth, the coming-out process can often either strengthen feelings of self-worth and safe dependence on caregivers or weaken attachment bonds. The practitioner can model activities to communicate enjoyment in connection and loving care to help repair potential distrust or hurt that may result from experienced LGBTQ stigma.

The practitioner can further strengthen engaging and nurturing activities by incorporating affirmative language into play. For example, the practitioner can help caregivers to lovingly "paint" their LGTBQ child's face with a feather, with affirmative narrations, such as "I'm coming to your sweet, soft cheek. This sweet, soft cheek is just right. Every part of you is just right!" LGBTQ caregivers may not necessarily need nurture and engagement to the extent that LGBTQ youth often do, although the practitioner can offer support through affirmative language to communicate that the LGBTQ family is just right. For example, the practitioner may incorporate structure with engagement and nurture to measure the family's hug and notice how strong their hugs are and how that family is just right as they are.

The following case illustration demonstrates how Theraplay can be adapted for intervention with a LGBTQ youth.

 ## CASE ILLUSTRATION
BRIEF CASE BACKGROUND

Kylie was a white, 12-year-old transgender girl (assigned male at birth but identifying as female) who was referred for therapy due to significant gender dysphoria that manifested as severe depression. Kylie had two white, cisgender, heterosexual parents named Lisa and Robert. Her parents were struggling to accept Kylie and had previously communicated that they thought her gender identity was a phase.

Kylie had become increasingly depressed in the last year as she had begun puberty. Her gender dysphoria had increased as her body had become more masculinized and she had become more withdrawn.

SESSION 1
During the first session, I met alone with Lisa and Robert to collect information about the family. I enquired about Kylie's developmental history and stressors, and their concerns and hopes for Kylie and their family. I also attended to Kylie's coming-out story, how she and her parents learned about her gender identity and how important people in her life had responded to her disclosure. Given that the disclosure process could potentially have been experienced as an attachment wound, I interviewed her parents carefully. I continued to assess for ways in which I could help the family strengthen attachment bonds. I prepared Lisa and Robert for Theraplay and they discussed how to introduce the MIM assessment to Kylie.

SESSIONS 2–3
I began the MIM session with Kylie, Lisa and Robert by introducing my social location (white, cisgender female, pansexual, etc.) and shared my stance as an affirmative practitioner. I asked Kylie for her preferred name and pronouns and emphasized the importance of creating a safe space together in session. The remainder of the second and third sessions was spent conducting the MIM for each parent. I assessed for strengths, areas for improvement and Kylie's attachment needs based on the Theraplay dimensions.

SESSION 4
During the fourth session, I met with Lisa and Robert and shared feedback, based on their MIM. I used psychoeducation about the dimensions of Theraplay and affirmed each parent's strengths. I was transparent about how I would refer to their child as "Kylie" and with "she/her" pronouns, as Kylie requested, even though the caregivers still struggle to use Kylie's preferred name and pronouns.

I emphasized that LGBTQ stigma may compound the gender dysphoria Kylie was experiencing. I was careful to avoid blaming them for their responses to Kylie's coming out and acknowledged their efforts to show love and support. I shared the importance of attending to minority stress and attachment to alleviate gender dysphoria and depression. I asked if I could continue to share information about best practices for helping TGD youth feel supported. I was transparent about my goals to increase Kylie's feelings of worth and safety with her caregivers and to support each caregiver by providing a safe space to process their feelings. I continued to frame the feedback session around the family's strengths and areas for growth. Together, we collaborated to construct a treatment plan based on their needs. Due to Lisa and Robert's reticence to engage with Kylie as their daughter, they decided to observe the next four sessions and continue to process their feelings and observations during consultation sessions.

SESSIONS 5–8
For the next four weeks, I conducted Theraplay sessions with Kylie while her parents observed interactions that promoted attunement. During these weeks, I also held weekly consultation sessions with the parents where I helped Lisa and Robert process their ambiguous loss about their perceptions of losing their son and gaining a daughter. I continued to weave psychoeducation about Theraplay and the impact of minority stress into these sessions to help them understand how they could better attune to Kylie. As these sessions progressed, Kylie's parents became more able to make decisions as a family about transitioning and to support Kylie. I continued to support the family and waited until all parties were ready for family sessions.

SESSIONS 9–18+
I led the sessions to promote attachment, helping the parents notice moments in which Kylie felt particularly cared for. Based on Kylie's needs, I emphasized engagement and nurture to increase feelings of safety, self-worth and mutual attunement. During these sessions, I wove affirmative language into play to model to Lisa and Robert how to attune to Kylie. For example, the adults initiated a blanket swing in which we sang, "Twinkle, twinkle, Kylie star; What a special girl you are! Golden hair and rosy cheeks; Big blue eyes from which you peek; Twinkle, twinkle, Kylie star; What a special girl you are!" Due to the degree of Kylie's gender dysphoria, I was careful when introducing activities that drew attention to her body. I helped Lisa and Robert balance structure and nurture when any activities revolved around awareness of her

body and coached them during consultation sessions to respond with openness, empathy and support if Kylie expressed dysphoric feelings about her body. I first guided Kylie's parents in activities that promoted nurturing engagement and affirmation around non-gendered body parts, such as initiating lotion and power prints and giving Kylie a manicure in session and highlighting how lovely her hands looked. I was careful to affirm non-gendered body parts (e.g., "Kylie, you had such strong breaths during that cotton ball race!") and was cautious about affirming any parts that could trigger gender dysphoria. For example, I affirmed Kylie's effort during a newspaper punch, rather than her strong arms, knowing that Kylie was dysphoric about the increases in muscle mass she had accumulated with puberty.

As the sessions progressed and Lisa and Robert gained more knowledge about Kylie's needs and became more prepared to meet these needs, they got increasingly more involved, under my guidance. I continued to meet with Lisa and Robert for consultation sessions every two to three sessions to highlight the family's growth and to help them continue to process difficulties that arose in parenting. I also normalized potential resistance and continued to use psychoeducation about Theraplay.

When working with TGD youth and families, the practitioner is often responsible for writing letters of support for social, legal and/or medical transitions, if the family needs this service. During treatment, I also met with the family to discuss Kylie's desires for transition. While all TGD people transition differently (or potentially not at all), Kylie and her parents decided that starting testosterone suppression hormones, followed by hormone replacement therapy, would be the best fit for her. Through therapy, Lisa and Robert became aware of the importance of supporting Kylie's transition in conjunction with creating positive attachment experiences to treat her gender dysphoria and depression. I wrote a letter for Kylie's medical doctor, confirming their treatment and my support for Kylie's transition. Theraplay sessions were terminated once Kylie's distress had significantly decreased, her parents felt confident in their abilities to respond to her needs, and the family had strengthened attachment bonds.

Conclusion

This chapter has provided an overview of the impact of minority stress on attachment bonds and how to integrate affirmative principles into Theraplay with LGBTQ families. While this chapter has presented suggestions for adaptations to Theraplay, the exact Theraplay sequences will vary based on each family member's needs, the degree of internalized stigma, and various contextual factors that interact with LGBTQ identities and may compound experiences with marginalization (e.g., race, ethnicity, religion, socio-economic status).

While this chapter has focused on LGBTQ families, it is important to remember that the families' gender identities and sexual orientations are not the only salient aspects of their identity. Thus, the practitioner needs to balance affirmation for LGBTQ identities and advocacy for the family with attending to other important aspects of who the clients are. To many in the community, they might be only known as "the only gay couple in the neighborhood" or "that one family with the LGBTQ child," so make sure to treat the family as whole and complete.

Questions for reflection and continued learning

1. Consider and discuss how you might apply the principles from this chapter to intervene with the following case with a child with LGBTQ parents.

   An LGBTQ family refer themselves to your office for family therapy. The family is composed of Jared (age nine) and two lesbian mothers, Julia (age 36), who is Jared's biological mother, and Jared's new stepmother, Ella (age 38). Julia divorced Jared's other mother, Teagan, several years ago due to "irreconcilable conflict." Jared has always been a healthy and happy child until the divorce. Recently, he has become more anxious and clingier in his relationship with Julia, especially since Julia has re-partnered with Ella. While Ella tries her best to have a connection with Jared, the mothers worry that Jared blames Ella for the divorce. Jared is struggling to develop a positive bond with Ella and has outbursts at home. Jared has been more withdrawn and defiant in the last few months. Julia also reports having been estranged from her family since she entered into a relationship with a woman.

2. Consider and discuss how you might apply the principles from this chapter to intervene with the following case with a child with LGBTQ adoptive parents.

   Matthew (age 34), Jonathan (age 32) and Tiana (age four) have referred themselves to your office for family therapy. Matthew and Jonathan are a married couple and have been together for the past seven years. The couple has wanted to become parents for some time and adopted Tiana 11 months ago. Matthew and Jonathan report that while their family is full of love, the road towards adoption has been full of obstacles. Matthew and Jonathan experienced numerous challenges, such as homophobic reactions from certain adoption agencies, microaggressions when trying to access support services (e.g., "Who is the real dad?"), and relational strain in their families of origin. While Matthew's parents fully support their marriage and the adoption of Tiana, Jonathan's father has not spoken to him since he and Matthew became engaged, and his mother does not fully support the relationship due to religious values. On top of these stressors, the couple reports feeling anxious about representing LGBTQ parents in a positive light. While Tiana seems to be adjusting well to her adoption, she is experiencing some difficulties related to verbal abuse she experienced from her birth family. Tiana experiences elevated anxiety and is very afraid of being separated from her fathers. The family is seeking support to help Tiana with her anxiety and to build more secure attachment bonds.

3. What have your experiences been in clinically intervening with LGBTQ families? What are your areas for growth to improve your clinical work with this population, in terms of potential biases, assumptions and your level of affirmative training? What additional resources might be of importance to LGBTQ families you might work with in your geographic area (e.g., PFLAG meetings, LGBTQ-affirmative churches, connections to TGD-affirmative endocrinologists, etc.)?

References

Bernal, A.T. & Coolhart, D. (2012). "Treatment and ethical considerations with transgender children and youth in family therapy." *Journal of Family Psychotherapy, 23*, 287–303. doi:10.1080/08975353.2012.735594.

Centers for Disease Control and Prevention. (2017). *Youth Risk Behavior Survey Questionnaire*. Retrieved from www.cdc.gov/yrbs.

Coolhart, D. (2012). "Supporting Transgender Youth and their Families in Therapy: Facing Challenges and Harnessing Strengths." In J. Bigner & J. Wetchler (eds) *Handbook of LGBT-Affirmative Couple and Family Therapy*. New York, NY: Routledge.

DeCamp, W. & Bakken, N.W. (2016). "Self-injury, suicide ideation, and sexual orientation: Differences in causes and correlates among high school students." *Journal of Injury and Violence Research, 8*(1), 15–23.

Drescher, J. & Byne, W. (2012). "Gender dysphoric/gender variant (GD/GV) children and adolescents: Summarizing what we know and what we have yet to learn." *Journal of Homosexuality, 59*, 501–510. doi:10.1080/00918369.2012.653317.

Harvey, R.G. & Stone Fish, L. (2015). "Queer youth in family therapy." *Family Process, 54*, 396–417. doi:10.1111/famp.12170.

House, A.S., Van Horn, E., Coppeans, C. & Stepleman, L.M. (2011). "Interpersonal trauma and discriminatory events as predictors of suicidal and nonsuicidal self-injury in gay, lesbian, bisexual, and transgender persons." *Traumatology, 17*(2), 75–78.

Levy, S.A., Russon, J. & Diamond, G.M. (2016). "Attachment-based family therapy for suicidal lesbian, gay, and bisexual adolescents: A case study." *Australian & New Zealand Journal of Family Therapy, 37*, 190–206. doi:10.1002/anzf.1151.

Manning, W.D., Fettro, M.N. & Lamidi, E. (2014). "Child well-being in same-sex parent families: Review of research prepared for American Sociological Association Amicus Brief." *Population Research and Policy Review, 33*, 485–502. doi:10.1007/s11113-014-9329-6.

Meyer, I.H. (2003). "Prejudice, social stress, and mental health in lesbian, gay, and bisexual populations: Conceptual issues and research evidence." *Psychological Bulletin, 129*, 674–697. https://doi.org/10.1037/0033-2909.129.5.674.

Meyer, I.H., Teylan, M. & Schwartz, S. (2015). "The role of help-seeking in preventing suicide attempts among lesbians, gay men, and bisexuals." *Suicide and Life-Threatening Behavior, 45*(1), 24–36.

Muehlenkamp, J., Hilt, L., Ehlinger, P. & McMillan, T. (2015). "Nonsuicidal self-injury in sexual minority college students: A test of theoretical integration." *Child and Adolescent Psychiatry Mental Health, 9*(16), 1–8.

Norwood, K. (2013). "Grieving gender: Trans-identities, transition, and ambiguous loss." *Communication Monographs, 80*, 24–45. doi:10.1080/03637751.2012.739705.

Pitoňák, M. (2017). "Mental health in non-heterosexuals: Minority stress theory and related explanation frameworks review." *Mental Health and Prevention, 5*, 63–73.

Rosario, M., Reisner, S.L., Corliss, H.L., Wypij, D., Frazier, A.L. & Austin, S.B. (2014). "Disparities in depressive distress by sexual orientation in emerging adults: The roles of attachment and stress paradigms." *Archives of Sexual Behavior, 43*, 901–916. doi:10.1007/s10508-013-0129-6.

Ryan, C. (2009). *Supporting Families, Healthy Children: Helping Families with Lesbian, Gay, Bisexual, & Transgender Children*. San Francisco, CA: Family Acceptance Project.

Smithee, L.C., Sumner, B.W. & Bean, R.A. (2019). "Non-suicidal self-injury among sexual minority youth: An etiological and treatment overview." *Children and Youth Services Review, 96*, 212–219. doi:10.1016/j.childyouth.2018.11.055.

Steensma, T.D., Biemond, R., de Boer, F. & Cohen-Kettenis, P.T. (2011). "Desisting and persisting gender dysphoria after childhood: A qualitative follow-up study." *Clinical Child Psychology and Psychiatry, 16*, 499–516. doi:10.1177/1359104510378303.

Trub, L., Quinlan, E., Starks, T.J. & Rosenthal, L. (2016). "Discrimination, internalized homonegativity, and attitudes toward children of same-sex parents: Can secure attachment buffer against stigma internalization?" *Family Process, 56*, 701–715. doi:10.1111/famp.12255.

World Professional Association for Transgender Health. (2018). *Standards of Care for the Health of Transsexual, Transgender, and Gender Nonconforming People* (seventh edition). Retrieved from www.wpath.org/media/cms/Documents/SOC%20v7/SOC%20V7_English.pdf.

Glossary of LGBTQ terms

Asexual: Describes a person who does not feel sexual desire or attraction for others.

Bisexual: Describes a person who is sexually, emotionally or romantically attracted to both men and women, or to more than one gender, although not necessarily to the same extent or in the same way.

Cisgender: A person whose assigned sex at birth aligns with their gender identity.

Cisnormativity: The assumption that all people are cisgender and/or that being cisgender is the normal or default way of being.

Coming out: An LGBTQ+ person's process of acknowledging and accepting their sexual and/or gender identity and sharing their identity and/or experiences with others.

Gay: Describes a person who is sexually, emotionally or romantically attracted to people of the same gender.

Gender dysphoria: Emotional distress related to feelings of incongruence between one's internal sense of gender and anatomical sex characteristics and/or cultural gender expectations.

Gender expansive: Describes a person who expresses their gender identity through a more flexible and wider expression than is usually associated with the binary gender system.

Gender expression: The outward ways that an individual expresses their gender identity, generally through means such as clothing, hair, voice and behavior. Gender expression may or may not conform to social norms and assumptions about binary gender.

Gender fluid: Describes a person who does not identify with one fixed gender identity.

Gender identity: A person's internal sense of being male, female, in between or neither male nor female. A person's gender can be the same as their assigned sex at birth (in the case of cisgender people) or it can differ from their assigned sex at birth (in the case of transgender and gender-diverse people).

Gender non-conforming: Describes a person whose gender expression (dress or behavior) does not neatly conform to traditional, binary social expectations.

Gender queer: Describes a person who does not identify as either solely masculine or feminine and instead identifies either entirely outside either these categories, as both male and female, or somewhere in between.

Gender transition: Defined broadly as a person's process of developing and assuming a gender expression to match their gender identity. Transition may include physical, legal and social transitions and varies based on a person's unique gender experience.

Heteronormativity: The assumption that all individuals are heterosexual and/or that being heterosexual is the normal/default way of being.

Homophobia: Discrimination, hatred, fear or discomfort with someone due to their attraction to others of the same sex. Homophobic might describe the attitudes and beliefs of a person, a group of people, a set of laws or even an institution.

Intersex: Describes a variety of natural bodily variations that do not fit the typical definitions of male or female sex (e.g., variations in chromosomes, genitals, gonads, sex hormones). Some of these variations might not be physically apparent at all, while other variations might not be apparent until puberty.

Lesbian: A woman who is sexually, emotionally and romantically attracted to other women.

LGBTQ: An acronym for lesbian, gay, bisexual, transgender and queer.

Non-binary: Describes a person who does not identify exclusively as either female or male. Similar to people who are gender queer, a non-binary person may identify entirely outside the male-female binary, as both male and female, or somewhere in between.

Outing: Exposing or sharing someone's LGBTQ+ identity/identities to others without the LGBTQ+ person's knowledge and consent. Outing may have serious consequences for the LGBTQ+ person's emotional safety, physical safety, economic stability and overall well-being.

Pansexual: Describes a person who has the potential to be sexually, emotionally or romantically attracted to people of any gender, although not necessarily to the same extent or in the same way.

Queer: Describes a person who is attracted to a wide variety of gender identities and expressions (similar to bisexual or pansexual). Queer is also often used interchangeably to describe someone who identifies broadly under the LGBTQ+ umbrella.

Questioning: Describes someone who is currently exploring their gender identity and/or sexual orientation.

Same-gender loving: A term some people use instead of an identity label (e.g., lesbian, gay) to describe their love and attraction to others of the same gender.

Sex assigned at birth: The sex (female or male) that doctors assign to a child at birth, based on their external anatomy (e.g., appearance of genitals).

Sexual orientation: A person's sexual, emotional and romantic attraction to other people.

Transgender/trans: A person whose gender identity, or internal sense of being male, female, in between or neither male nor female, differs from the sex assigned to them at birth. Since gender is distinct from sexuality, being transgender does not imply the person's sexual orientation (straight, gay, lesbian, pansexual, bisexual).

Transphobia: Discrimination, hatred, fear or discomfort with someone due to their identification as transgender. Transphobic might describe the attitudes and beliefs of a person, a group of people, a set of laws or even an institution.

Adapted from https://www.hrc.org/resources/glossary-of-terms.

Chapter 12

Theraplay with Children who are Deaf or Hard of Hearing

Alexis Greeves and Nicki Melby

Introduction

Thirty-four million children around the world have some form of hearing loss (World Health Organization, 2019). How hearing loss affects relationships, educational opportunities and a sense of self will vary from individual to individual. What we do know is that many of these children may have limited access to mental health support or, at the very least, limited access to therapists who take into consideration how they may have a different experience than their hearing peers. Theraplay, as a mental health intervention, is an effective way of supporting the needs of these children when offered through a culturally competent lens and with an understanding of the unique experiences of the child with hearing loss. This chapter will explore the ways that Theraplay can be used to meet the needs of the children who are deaf or hard of hearing and their families. The following treatment example will set the stage for this discussion.

 Dominic and his mother enter the office together walking backwards, holding hands and laughing. As they sit down, side by side, I (Alexis Greeves) sign to Dominic, "BIG-SMILE BROUGHT TODAY." (Note: Capitalization of words indicates the signs the authors used in the syntax of American Sign Language.) He smiles at me and glances at his mom who then lovingly touches his dimples. "YES, DIMPLES TOO." I place a whale beanie baby on his head and sign, "I SAY 'WHALE,' YOU HEAD-FORWARD DROP." Dominic nods as I place the whale atop his head and then I sign, "YELLOW...SILLY...NEW YORK...WHALE!" (These are all signs that use the "y" handshape.) He drops the whale into my awaiting hands as Mom and I shake our hands back and forth over our heads as a form of light applause.

Dominic is seven years old, African American and deaf. His medical diagnosis is profound bilateral sensorineural hearing loss. Dominic also has a strong Deaf cultural identity. His primary language is American Sign Language (ASL); he attends a local school for the deaf where his peers, and the majority of his teachers, coaches, support staff and administration, are also deaf. His mother, however, struggles to communicate with him. Sara is hearing and had never met a deaf person prior to giving birth to her son. On learning of his hearing loss, Sara became depressed and distanced herself from her baby, overwhelmed with the idea of raising a child she thought of as "disabled." Dominic was fitted with hearing aids and Sara used speech and gestures to communicate with him. However, she realized that she spent most of her time teaching and correcting his speech, rather than enjoying him and accepting his deafness. Eventually, Sara moved her son to the local school for the deaf and found that her son began to thrive, both linguistically and in his social-emotional development. By the time he reached first grade, Sara could see that Dominic had a great passion for his place in school, but she felt distant from her son. At home, she noted that he would often get frustrated easily and didn't seek out her help. When she attempted to calm him down, he would become angry and at times aggressive with her. Sara wondered if her early depression at the time of her son's diagnosis may have caused a separation between the two of them. She went for counseling to help with this.

Key points

Dominic's story illustrates a number of the key points influencing the implementation of Theraplay for children with hearing loss:

1. Practitioners working with children with any degree of hearing loss must understand how those with hearing loss/their family members identify themselves and their culture. Individuals may identify as Deaf, deaf, having a degree of hearing loss, or hearing but with some loss. The differences will be discussed in this chapter.

2. Through the lens of Porges' (2018) polyvagal theory, we can better

understand a deaf child's struggle to seek social engagement from a caregiver who cannot communicate with him or her and the child's potential quick move into defensive fight, flight, freeze or collapse. This difficulty in the child's arousal regulation can lead to behavior and attachment difficulties.

3. Hearing caregivers of a deaf child may have unresolved grief from the diagnosis of their child's hearing loss. They may struggle to become attuned to the child's needs for regulation and connection. The caregivers' grief and struggles connecting and regulating also can lead to attachment difficulties. Theraplay offers an opportunity for these caregivers to have joyful interaction with their children and repair ruptures that may have resulted from disconnection as a result of grief and loss reactions.

4. Theraplay addresses both the arousal and attachment issues seen in families with children with hearing loss. Because the Theraplay model is not "language-heavy," it is an ideal intervention when there are differences in the language systems of the parent and child. For many deaf children with hearing caregivers, the differences are spoken English (hearing caregivers) and American Sign Language (for some deaf children).

5. Theraplay activities will need to be "tweaked" in order to become more "Deaf friendly" when working with children and families in which someone has a hearing loss.

The Deaf community

When I (Alexis Greeves) meet Deaf individuals in my work, one of the first questions I'm asked is what is my connection with the Deaf community—do I have parents or siblings who are deaf? Culturally, this is an important way of identifying to what degree I am an ally of the Deaf community. When referring to children with hearing loss, there is a range of descriptions—one being a child who identifies as culturally Deaf (signified by the capital "D"). The Deaf community is recognized as having a visual language, American Sign Language (ASL), that is differentiated in its vocabulary, syntax and grammar to a spoken language like English. This is also true of many other sign languages throughout the world—Kenyan Sign Language, Thai Sign Language and New Zealand Sign Language are examples of just a few. The Deaf community identifies as a linguistic minority, rather than individuals who have a disability. Deaf culture refers to art, storytelling, humor and communication norms that are unique to this group (We the Deaf People, 2016–2019). A Deaf child may have Deaf caregivers and their deafness is accepted and celebrated. A child may also identify as being deaf, having mild to significant hearing loss and perhaps uses hearing aids, cochlear implants or other devices to assist in communicating with hearing individuals. This child may not yet be exposed to the Deaf community or have met other deaf/Deaf people, potentially leaving them to feel they might be the only deaf person in their community or, in some cases, the only deaf person alive. Someone who is hard of hearing may identify as such or as being "hearing" but with some hearing loss.

American Deaf culture can be described as encompassing traditions, values and behaviors that center around American Sign Language and identifying with other Deaf individuals. Deaf culture can also include the value of an environment that promotes visual contact as well as strategies such as tapping on one's shoulder or turning lights on and off to get someone's attention. Within Deaf culture (as in many other cultures), there is a desire to see the culture thrive and continue on through generations. This desire may be carried out through stories, fables, visual poetry, art, dance, sports and opportunities for people to come together to celebrate en masse (Laurent Clerc National Deaf Education Center, 2015).

Theraplay with families wherein one or more members of the family is deaf or hard of hearing can be useful. I do want to note that as a hearing person, fluent in ASL, I write from my own experience of providing direct communication in my work. Many hearing therapists who may encounter a deaf client and don't have fluency in ASL will want to hire an ASL interpreter. I cannot speak about the experience of having an interpreter also present in the room. This may change the dynamic and slow down the process; however, I surmise that Theraplay can be equally effective as long as all parties are aware of their roles in the therapy space.

Problems in arousal

Children who are deaf and grow up in a home where communication is difficult may experience hyperarousal in response to lack of information.

For example, Dominic has a younger hearing sister, Klarissa. One day their parents are fighting in the kitchen while their two children are in the living room working on homework. Klarissa is bracing herself emotionally and in her nervous system as she hears her angry father exit the kitchen and approach them. She keeps her eyes on the page. Meanwhile, Dominic looks up and is eager to show his father what he's been working on, unaware of his father's distressed state. He approaches his father only to be yelled at (the words he's unsure of, but he certainly recognizes being scolded) and is left confused by what he has done to earn his father's ire.

Stephen Porges' polyvagal theory discusses the use of social engagement—the ability to create co-regulation and seeking out safety (Porges, 2018). Whereas Klarissa may seek out a parent to help her make sense of her feelings once the tension in the home is at rest, Dominic is left to experience the shame of having angered his father (in his mind) and not knowing who or how to seek out help. Porges' theory would suggest that enough of these interactions may render a child to move quickly from social engagement (remaining within their window of tolerance) to fight or flight. Even with an available, caring adult, if communication is strained or a child misreads a parent's facial expression ("Mom is so angry with me, I don't feel safe!"), the social engagement system may not be activated and again the child would move outside their window of tolerance and become withdrawn or aggressive. In working with these parents, it's important to build attunement to Dominic's experience and to his nervous system state. Whereas Klarissa seeks out connection, Dominic moves quickly into protection. Within Theraplay, it would be important for Dominic to experience joyful engagement with his parents, to experience time and again that his parents can be trusted to hold his emotions. In a parent consultation session, I encourage Dominic's parents to seek him out when he is outside his window of tolerance and to remain in his presence. Once he is more regulated, they are then to explain that his father had become angry in the midst of a discussion with Mom and that this has nothing to do with Dominic's behavior. It's important for Dominic's parents to recognize that what Klarissa as a hearing child takes in as incidental information ("my parents are arguing and I'd better give Dad his space"), Dominic doesn't have access to. He needs to be told, "Son, your mom and I are having a difficult discussion and I'm feeling upset. I need a few moments to take care of myself."

Unresolved grief of parents

The *Sesame Street* writer Emily Perl Kingsley wrote a short essay entitled *Welcome to Holland* in which she describes planning for a trip to Italy and landing in Holland (2019). This metaphor of her experience of having a child with Down syndrome gave a great deal of hope to caregivers grieving the discovery of a child with disabilities. Such is also the experience for many hearing families when they discover their child is born deaf. For most families, they have never encountered a deaf person, have minimal, if any, exposure to American Sign Language, and are grieving the loss of the child they thought would come into their lives. Approaching the medical establishment for help can also be overwhelming as suggestions of surgery and intensive forms of speech and hearing practice are recommended. Caregivers can feel lost, isolated and disconnected from their deaf baby as they navigate this new world, often without peers in their community to join or steer them.

While deaf caregivers of deaf children may also experience a form of grief, it's not usually met with the same level of shock, anger or confusion that hearing caregivers undergo. Deaf caregivers may feel a sense of ambivalence towards having a deaf child; they may grieve that their child may suffer the inequities and oppression that they experience living and working in a hearing world, while simultaneously be celebrating having a child who will adopt their cultural beliefs, mores and language.

For hearing caregivers unsure of how to bond with their deaf child, or who are seeking out therapy years after post-partum depression or a period of mourning the loss of the child they thought they would have, Theraplay sessions offer an opportunity for them to experience joyful connection and emotional attunement with their child. Theraplay offers a "do-over" for caregivers who feel as though the window has closed on the opportunity to bond with their child. Nurturing activities such as the blanket swing (imitating rocking an infant) or feeding (harking back to nursing or bottle feeding) provide the child and caregiver with the experiences that were missed.

Different language systems

Caregivers with minimal sign language skills can be at ease with games and activities that allow them to communicate through eye contact, touch, attunement and engagement. While it is my belief that it is in the best interest of sign language-using children for their caregivers to learn and become as fluent as possible in ASL, I also believe that we need to meet families where they are and minimize shame. Theraplay allows caregivers to communicate to their child their affection and their ability to create structure and intimacy as well as to hold the child's present moment experience. A number of children at schools for the deaf have hearing caregivers, and of those, many don't know more than a few functional signs.

While I was working as a school counselor at a school for the deaf, I helped host a gathering of caregivers and children in celebration of Valentine's Day. We set up several stations of Theraplay activities and invited caregivers to move through the stations with their children. At one station, we had several chairs in two rows facing one another. We invited a caregiver to sit on one side facing their child and offered each adult a cotton ball. The caregivers gently drew letters on their child's face, allowing the child to guess the letter, then eventually spelling out words like "love," "cute," "special" and the child's name. At another station, caregivers and children traced the child's hand in the shape of the "I Love You" handshape and wrote in each finger on the paper something special about their child. At another station, caregivers used toilet paper to wrap their child up like a mummy (with the child given the option of having their arms wrapped by their sides or unwrapped to allow them to sign). On the count of three, the child burst out of the mummy wrap to great celebration from the caregivers. This night was lauded as a great success and many caregivers stated how wonderful it was to engage with their child in a joyful way (Greeves, 2008).

Adapting Theraplay for deaf children

Some Theraplay activities may need to be adapted to make sense in ASL. For example, "Zoom-Erk" is a game used with words to "pass along" a zooming car that a member of the group can stop suddenly by "hitting on the brakes" and saying "ERK!" and then passing back the opposite direction by saying "Zoom!" while making eye contact with the person on the reverse side. When I play this with a family member who is deaf, we would sign a car going fast ("CAR GO ZOOM!") to the person to our left, for example, and when someone in the group wants to send it in the opposite direction, they would sign "CAR STOPPING SUDDENLY" and then looking at the person to their right sign "CAR GO ZOOM!"

In Theraplay games, when a "cue word" is given to indicate to the child to do something (i.e., in beanie baby drop or newspaper punch), the caregiver and therapist's hands may be occupied ready to catch the beanie baby or holding the newspaper taut. Rather than giving a cue word, the practitioner explains that when both her eyes suddenly shut tight, it's the cue for the child to drop the beanie baby or punch the newspaper. The practitioner may then wiggle her nose, wink one eye, wink another and then blink both eyes shut in an exaggerated form to indicate "Now!"

CASE ILLUSTRATIONS
ALEXIS'S CASE

Carter was a five-year-old, Caucasian boy born in the mid-Atlantic region of the US to hearing parents Susanne and Oliver. He was diagnosed with profound, sensorineural bilateral hearing loss soon after his newborn infant screening. The cause of this hearing loss is unknown. At the suggestion of the early intervention team, Carter's parents had decided to enroll their child in an early education center for deaf children, with a focus on using spoken language and listening (an "oral method"). After two years in this program, Carter's parents were noticing an increase in his frustration—Carter would often take off his hearing aids and throw them at his parents. He resorted to hitting and screaming rather than "using his words" to tell his parents what he wanted. He and his younger sister Annie had developed some homemade signs that allowed her to "translate" to her parents what she believed was upsetting her older brother. At the encouragement of some friends, Carter's parents explored and then started him at the local school for the deaf that used American Sign Language. Mom and Dad started meeting deaf adults for the first time and were taking their first class in ASL. The school social worker had referred them to my clinic to help with "controlling, non-compliant behaviors."

After the initial intake, I scheduled a Marschak Interaction Method assessment with each of the parents. On review, I observed that, for each of the parents, setting structure was a struggle. They would hand the envelopes with the props over to Carter and would read the card aloud while simultaneously scattering a few signs that didn't appear to make much sense to Carter. Aloud they would read, "Adult draws a picture and asks the child to draw one just like it." Signing Mom said, "Me [pointing at paper]. You [pointing at paper]." Carter nodded as if to indicate that he understood; however, I surmised that he had become accustomed to nodding to his mother to keep communication moving along and to appease her, rather than indicating that he didn't understand.

When the MIM card stated that the adult leaves the room without the child, Dad had stood up and patted the table and signed "stay" to Carter and walked out the door. The video showed that Carter stared at the door with his hands moving back and forth on the table in an effort to soothe himself; he then became very still and appeared to dissociate. When Dad returned, he smiled weakly at Carter and picked up the next card and moved on with the assessment.

In our family feedback session, I noted that while it was evident to me that, yes, Carter was often attempting to wrest control from his parents, it was most likely driven by fear and confusion. From all reports, Carter was a clever and curious child and was aware of events happening around him but was often confused by why they were happening. He was also attuned enough to know that his hearing, younger sister had more access to information than he did and was at times resentful of her while simultaneously dependent on her to help him make sense of events. The following is an example that I explored with his parents in order to help us make sense of his experiences.

Carter and Annie were sitting at the kitchen table on a Friday afternoon enjoying a snack. Mom was on the phone with a friend telling her that the following day, Saturday, she would be dropping off the children at Grandma's house so that she, Mom, could go buy a gift for her nephew. Annie then had incidental information that Carter didn't have. The following morning, Mom quickly told the children to hop in the car. To Annie she said, "Hop in the car, honey! We're going to Grandma's!" To Carter she signed, "CAR NOW PLEASE." Carter looked out of the window wondering where they were going. Would it be somewhere fun? Or could it be scary, like the doctor's office? He was unsure and smiled tentatively at his sister as she played calmly with a doll she had brought with her. Shortly, he recognized the street they were turning onto as his grandmother's and, for the first time since getting in the car, his anxiety about their destination finally started to dissipate. This experience happened again the following day when they set off for their cousin's birthday party, Annie knowing where they were going and Carter once again anxious and unsure of where he was heading and why.

Exploring Carter's experience of the world through the lens of his deafness helped his parents better understand why he might feel a need to control his environment. I also explained that, despite this maladaptive need, Carter continued to look to his parents to interpret the world and his experiences for him. While watching the MIM, we observed the many moments that Carter looked up at his parents for confirmation and encouragement.

Mom proved to be strong in the nurture dimension, while this was a struggle for Dad. Both parents proved to have difficulty in the dimension of engagement. These would then become the areas of focus for our Theraplay work. We agreed that I would work primarily with Mom and Carter to begin with as she had more flexibility to come in and we would shift to bringing Dad in at a later date.

At our first session, I had Carter and Mom take five giant steps into the room and then plop down side by side on the bean-bag cushion. I signed without using my voice to Carter that I was so pleased to see him and that I saw he brought his big brown eyes with him. I checked in with Mom to see if she was following my signs and she nodded, so I proceeded to ask Mom in ASL what she noticed Carter had brought with him. She pointed at his smile while she also smiled and I signed, "YES! HIS BIG SMILE!!"

I then plopped a monkey beanie baby on my head and held Carter's hands together in front of me while bowing my head to allow the monkey to fall off and into Carter's hands. He laughed and as he attempted to throw it towards Mom, I took his hands in mine and gently placed the monkey on his head. I told him that, when he saw my eyes do a big blink, to drop the monkey into my hands. He looked closely into my eyes and, after seeing my blink, nodded his head and allowed the monkey to fall into my hands. After doing this a few times, I asked him if I could see his strong arm muscle. He proudly showed me his five-year-old bicep and Mom and I showed an exaggerated "Wow!" facial expression. I demonstrated to Mom the sign for "Wow" and encouraged her to sign it as well. I then showed him my "karate hand" and asked if he had one too. He showed it to me and again Mom signed "Wow!" I explained that Mom and I would be holding some crepe paper taut in front of him and when I signed "blue" he could chop through the paper. I signed "RED," "GREEN" and "BLUE" and his little hand chopped through the paper. He puffed out his chest and I turned to Mom and said while signing, "Look how proud he is!" Mom signed back, "I'm proud too!" At the end of this session I had Mom feed Carter some fruit snacks. He attempted to take the fruit snacks in his hand to feed himself. I gently took his hand and said, "Mom would love to feed you," and Mom proceeded to feed him.

Sessions continued with me introducing activities, and then over time, as Mom became more comfortable and skilled, I slowly had her lead the activities. One of Mom and Carter's favorite activities was the magic carpet. Carter sat on a folded blanket and Mom held two corners. When Carter made eye contact with Mom, she would move the "carpet" around the room. When he looked away she stopped until he gazed into her eyes again. Initially he would avoid eye contact, but as he started to enjoy the experience of moving around the room, he held eye contact longer. Mom would then sometimes make goofy faces that had them both laughing.

Mom later reported that as she spent more time in Theraplay sessions, she felt more attuned to Carter's needs. At home, she began to notice his behaviors in a new light and saw his actions as communication, rather than "acting out." As each parent became comfortable with the Theraplay activities in sessions, they integrated the activities into daily routines at home. At night, Carter would sit on his bed facing his mother as his father sat behind him. Dad would do a weather report on his back, patting his fingers over Carter's back while his mother would sign "RAINING OUTSIDE," and then when Mom would sign "THUNDERSTORM" Dad would make fists and massage his son's back until Mom signed "MOON APPEAR" and he would gently make smoothing motions over the whole of his back. The family came to delight in these times together and they experienced connection beyond what they had before.

NICKI'S CASE

Lulu was a deaf 11-year-old girl whose family immigrated from Laos when she was seven years old. Lulu was never exposed to formal language before coming to America. She only communicated with her mother through gestures and pointing to things. After arriving in the United States, Lulu was mainstreamed with other hearing children at a local public school with the assistance of American Sign Language interpreters. As Lulu started to pick up sign language, she also became aggressive toward her mother. Lulu's aggression would escalate to a point that her mother feared for her safety. Lulu's family did not sign or speak English. A deaf and hard of hearing teacher from her school referred Lulu to therapy due to her mother's concerns about Lulu's threatening behaviors.

When I met Lulu and her mother for the first time, Lulu reported that she did not believe that her mother loved her and that her mother always seemed to be angry, stating that her mother always "made angry facial expressions." I decided to use Theraplay as an intervention to improve the mother-daughter relationship, especially as there was no formal language present. I started by modeling Theraplay activities with Lulu, then had Mom do the activities with her.

I gestured to Mom "watch us" and did a hand stack with Lulu. After this, I invited Mom to try and she immediately joined in. Lulu and her mother both giggled as they lay hands on top of one another. Holding a cotton ball, I then explained to Lulu that I would make a pretend painting on her arm and asked what picture she wanted painted. She signed "BUTTERFLY" and I drew a picture of a butterfly for Mom, and then while the mother watched me, I painted on Lulu's arm a picture of a butterfly. Mom then followed my lead by asking Lulu what Mom could draw and Mom followed suit, painting it on her daughter's arm.

During the painting activity, both made eye contact and smiled at each other. Mom gestured with both of her hands on the middle of her chest, showing her daughter her love for her, which Lulu smiled back. In subsequent sessions, the mother-daughter duo did activities together with more independence from me and their relationship improved significantly. Mom reported that Lulu became more loving and less threatening towards her.

This case illustration shows that even when there is a language barrier, loving and enjoyable relationships between parents and child are possible.

Other considerations

Because of the lack of mental health resources available in most areas for deaf clients, many times they are referred to hearing practitioners who have had minimal to no experience working with this population. We believe it is the ethical responsibility of these practitioners to explore if there is a practitioner in the area who is fluent in American Sign Language (if that is the preferred communication choice of the client) and is aware of the specific needs of the client with a hearing loss. Having taken an ASL class and knowing fingerspelling (spelling out letters in ASL to form English words) does not make one proficient enough to work with a deaf client. If there isn't a practitioner in your community who is fluent in ASL, let the referred client know that you will work alongside a certified ASL interpreter to provide your services. There are resources to help practitioners best understand how to work alongside an interpreter for best results (e.g., Kirkpatrick, 2016).

Many communities may not have certified interpreters or the practitioner may not be in a position to work alongside an interpreter. Theraplay can also be successful if the focus is on non-verbal Theraplay activities. The practitioner's focus is to keep the child within his/her window of tolerance, which would mean the onus is on the practitioner to follow the child's language needs, and not to encourage the child to speak (unless that is the child's preference) or to sign (unless that is the child's preference). It is also our belief that the practitioner should seek consultation from a Theraplay-trained practitioner who has experience working with the Deaf population to ascertain specific activities adapted for deaf children, as well as to answer questions that arise about cultural competency or potential countertransference.

Conclusion

Theraplay is indeed a powerful modality that can be used successfully in families with deaf children or children with any level of hearing loss, whether the child identifies as culturally Deaf or not. The secure and attuned caregiver can help their child access social engagement and keep him/her from moving into fight, flight, freeze or collapse. For some caregivers, their unresolved grief may prevent them from being attuned to the child's needs, and these caregivers will need healing from their own pain before turning to their child's. For caregivers who don't have strong signing skills, Theraplay provides a means of connecting with their child through nurturing touch, eye contact and playful activities. Through Theraplay, caregivers are given a shame-free space to become attuned to their child and as a result can respond as any caregiver would want to—with structure, affection and delight.

Questions for reflection and continued learning

1. What are some reasons for using Theraplay when there is a language difference between caregiver and child, and specifically if one of them is deaf?

2. What modifications can you make to some Theraplay activities that will allow for attunement if there is a language discrepancy between parent and child?

3. Why would it be important to talk to hearing parents of deaf children about their possible "lack of incidental information"?

References

Greeves, A. (2008, Winter). "Theraplay with deaf children and hearing parents." *The Theraplay Institute Newsletter.*

Kirkpatrick, K. (2016). *Ten Tips for Using a Sign Language Interpreter.* National Institutes of Health Office of Equity, Diversity and Inclusion. Retrieved from www.edi.nih.gov/blog/communities/10-tips-using-sign-language-interpreter.

Laurent Clerc National Deaf Education Center. (2015). *American Deaf Culture.* Retrieved from www3.gallaudet.edu/clerc-center/info-to-go/deaf-culture/american-deaf-culture.html.

Pearl Kingsley, E. (2019). *A Parent's Perspective: Welcome to Holland.* Retrieved from www.ndss.org/resources/a-parents-perspective.

Porges, S.W. (2018). "Polyvagal Theory: A Primer." In S.W. Porges & D. Dana (eds) *Clinical Applications of the Polyvagal Theory* (pp.50–69). New York, NY: W.W. Norton & Company.

We the Deaf People. (2016–2019). *Deaf People as Linguistic Minority.* Retrieved from www.wtdp.org/preview/position-statements/15-deaf-people-as-a-lingusitic-minority.

World Health Organization. (2019, March 20). *Deafness and Hearing Loss.* Retrieved from www.who.int/news-room/fact-sheets/detail/deafness-and-hearing-loss.

Subject Index

Author Index

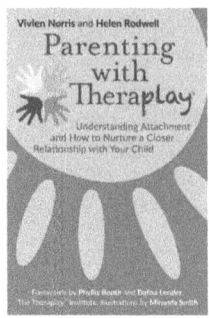

Parenting with Theraplay®
Understanding Attachment and How to Nurture a Closer Relationship with Your Child
Dr. Vivien Norris and Dr. Helen Rodwell

Paperback: £13.99/$19.95
ISBN: 978 1 78592 209 1
eISBN: 978 1 78450 489 2
208 pages

Theraplay® is an attachment-focused model of parenting that helps parents to understand and relate to their child. Based on a sequence of play activities that are rooted in neuroscience, Theraplay offers a fun and easy way for parents and children to connect. Theraplay is particularly effective with looked-after and adopted children.

As it provides an overview of Theraplay and the psychological principles that it is based on, parents and carers will gain an understanding of the basic theory of the model along with practical ideas for applying Theraplay to everyday family life. Through everyday case studies and easy language, parents will gain confidence and learn new skills for emotional bonding, empathy and acceptance in the relationship with their child.

· ·

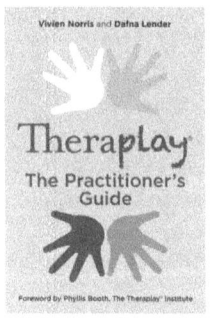

Theraplay®
The Practitioner's Guide
Dr. Vivien Norris and Dafna Lender

Paperback: £27.99/$34.95
ISBN: 978 1 78592 210 7
eISBN: 978 1 78450 488 5
392 pages

The definitive guide to Theraplay® for practitioners, officially endorsed by The Theraplay® Institute.

This comprehensive guide outlines the theory, reflection and skill development of the practitioner—the true power house of Theraplay. By maintaining a focus on practice throughout, embedding theory into practice examples, it brings the spirit of Theraplay to life. Part 1 covers the key principles of the intervention; Part 2 addresses Theraplay in practice: how to use the Marschak Interaction Method (MIM), how to set up a room and choose activities and considerations for working with different client groups; Part 3 encourages the reader to engage in their own development and the stages involved; and Parts 4 and 5 provide a wealth of useful resources, checklists, handouts, sample sessions and an up-to-date list of Theraplay activities.